Integrative Healing

Taking the CAM therapists' game
up a notch. A practical, common sense
guide for creating a more professional look.

Integrative Healing

Taking the CAM therapists' game
up a notch. A practical, common sense
guide for creating a more professional look.

Lorinda Weatherall

AYNI
BOOKS

Winchester, UK
Washington, USA

First published by Ayni Books, 2012
Ayni Books is an imprint of John Hunt Publishing Ltd., Laurel House, Station Approach,
Alresford, Hants, SO24 9JH, UK
office1@o-books.net
www.o-books.com

For distributor details and how to order please visit the 'Ordering' section on our website.

Text copyright: Lorinda Weatherall 2011

ISBN: 978 1 84694 963 0

A CIP catalogue record for this book is available from the British Library.

Design: Stuart Davies

Printed and bound by CPI Group (UK) Ltd, Croydon, CR0 4YY

We operate a distinctive and ethical publishing philosophy in all
areas of our business, from our global network of authors to
production and worldwide distribution.

CONTENTS

Preface

The journey was started by an invitation to attend a local children's playgroup, when my youngest son was not yet 3 and I had never heard of Reiki. If someone had told me that this synchronicity would lead to writing a Reiki manual to help the public and the medical community co-operate with one another, I would have laughed.

Not because the idea was not a good one. Oh no, by all means, it is an excellent idea. But it would be more of 'Why me?' The next question might have been "Why not you?"

So here we are 17+ years later, my son has become an adult and I am eager to facilitate this evolving mass of potential that is in Healthcare.

Modern medicine has done its very best trying to assist the many billions of us who inhabit this planet to live long, healthy and productive lives. But it wasn't always this way.

Scientists discovered that when they looked at a sample of our world underneath a microscope it was very different than this one and quite scary. They discovered that it was inhabited by bacteria, viruses, parasites, protozoa etc. Researchers also discovered that there were good and bad organisms in this microscopic world.

For example there are good (Acidophilus) and bad (E. coli) strains of bacteria. The good strains make blue cheese but the bad ones are nasty and make people sick.

Viennese Doctor Ingaz Semmelweis realized this in 1840. Semmelweis theorized and then proved that if doctors washed their hands after examining corpses in the morgue before seeing women in the obstetrics ward, these women did not contract childbed fever nor did they subsequently die. Unfortunately, his colleagues did not share his point of view.

A scant 40 years later Louis Pasteur discovered the existence of microscopic organisms. This discovery forced doctors to recognize the need for cleanliness and antiseptic conditions.[1]

Traditional healing spots are known all over the world, I am sure you could name a few. Whether it is taking the mineral baths in Germany, Banff, Alberta or even the healing waters at Lourdes, France.

Is it a matter of faith? Sometimes. Is it the fervent belief in a Supreme Being or a Saint; could it be sheer willpower on behalf of the one who is sick? Could be, but in any case they get better.

Our past is filled with stories - folklore and old wives' tales of men and women who had "the gift" or to some it may have been a curse. These were men and women who lived quietly amongst their communities but were sought out when someone was sick because they knew how to heal.

How and why these healings happened we are not exactly sure, but we do know that healing did happen.

Now add to this mix of medicine and unexplained healing the realm of Quantum physics. The Quantum world may not solve or answer all our questions but, just as our world was changed over a hundred years ago by the discovery of the microscope, things are about to get a whole lot smaller.

This manual is not a science book filled with all kinds of Quantum equations, nor is it a book filled with nebulous concepts.

A quick search of the internet (2010) shows that over 84 medical schools in the United States are offering some courses in Complementary Therapies.

Due to patient driven questioning of their General Practitioners [in the United States], some the medical schools in the U.S. have decided to include courses in Complementary and Alternative Medicine. (CAM):

Public interest in and use of complementary and alternative therapies continue to grow. Given this interest, we feel that family physicians have a responsibility to their patients to develop a basic understanding of the principles and applications of CAM in primary care.

No standardized curriculum is available for medical educators in this field. Providing an adequate background on these therapies and reliable, useful information to our learners was a task addressed by the Society of Teachers of Family Medicine (STFM) Group on Alternative Medicine over the past 2 years. [1999]

The recommended guidelines should serve as an aid to family practice residencies undertaking the challenge of integrating teaching on complementary and alternative therapies into their curricula.[1]

Once you know the language, we are not so different after all. Based upon the guidelines [which are provided in the Appendix] these Doctors have to learn—in my humble view—we in the Complementary field have to take our game up a notch, so to speak.

It is my hope that this book is a starting point for dialog between the healers and those who work in modern medicine.Integrative Healing: Merging with Modern Medicine is not just for people who are Reiki practitioners who want to share their talents with clients in the allopathic medicine field. But a guide for anyone and any modality in the Complementary field.

Here is a brief history about me, and how this all fits together.

As a small child my family often remarked how caring and compassionate I was about other living things, birds, my cat and other people. They suggested that I get involved in nursing or become a veterinarian. While those are good career choices, I wanted to do something different.

I chose Physical Anthropology, which is the study of humans through the physical remains. This covers a wide time span, from the first hominid remains around 4.4 million years ago, right up to now, including forensic science. This was before DNA technology and the TV show CSI. The course requirements meant learning some anatomy (bones, muscles, etc) and some pathology (leprosy, arthritis, tooth decay) and a little statistics to figure out stature and weight. Sometimes we used preserved primate specimens but most times we had human resin skeletons to look at.

My passion with Reiki started in 1994 with my first teacher Nancy L. Bradley. The day was quite uneventful really. There were 8 people in the class, some were more energy sensitive than I was, but that did not stop me from working on myself or on my young family.

Initially, I was only interested in the beginner's class. However, within 6 months I signed up for the middle class – Level 2. In August of 1996, I fully embraced the title of Reiki Master or Teacher, and I stepped onto the road that has led me to this point.

Should you discover any errors or omissions while reading this material, I apologize for the errors; and like a good editor I welcome your suggestions.

I would like to offer a heartfelt thanks to Nicole B. now H. for that invitation; my life would not be the same if I had not met you. And a hearty thanks to all the health loving friends and clients I have had along the way. To all my teachers, thank you for your encouragement, enlightenment and wisdom.

When contemplating sitting down and assembling this manual it always came down to where do I start and how do I go about putting it together. By the grace of the Internet I discovered a wonderful site www.iteckworld.co.uk in England that gave quite a detailed Reiki Syllabus.

This site by sharing their outline assisted in fleshing out and bringing to life Integrative Healing. I am thoroughly grateful to ITEC for your attention to detail and wish you success at all your teaching locations.

Thank you to John H. at O-Books for seeing the value of this subject, and my initial contact Pauline C. at Anyi who felt that the material contained within these pages would appeal to a wider audience. Finally, the editing department Susannah, Trevor and others for your editing expertise and valued assistance.

Last but not least my family and extended family for their understanding when I rave on about energy healing and science stuff. I hope I have not injured you too badly due to the intensity or insanity with which I have examined this subject.

Yours in Health, Lorinda Weatherall
Written 25th April 2013.

Chapter 1

Energy Medicine

What is it?

Energy Medicine is the name given to a group of healing therapies (modalities), which use or interact with the subtle energies of the body or the biofield. Acupuncture, Esoteric Healing, Homeopathy, Polarity Balancing, Pranic Healing, Qi Gong, Reiki and Therapeutic Touch are just a few.

For example: When we rub the anterior surface (palms) of our hands together, in most cases they get warm. If you were to open your hands 4 or 5 inches (10 to 12.5 cm) apart you might feel some resistance. Almost as if there was an invisible ball in between your palms.

That is subtle energy or the subtle energy field.

Now take one of your palms (right or left hand) and slowly move it over the opposite arm. Did you feel anything? Was there warmth, or were the hairs on your arm standing on edge? Did it feel cool or like a damp breeze?

This is also subtle energy, your biofield.

Each human on the planet has it, however if you were to question each person would they be aware of it? Or would we even call it the same thing?

The human body has a subtle energy system that interpenetrates the physical anatomy and extends outward beyond it.

Disease or disorder can be detected in the energy system (perhaps before it manifests in the physical body) and can be affected therapeutically by the action of energy practitioners, in support of the self-healing capacity of the body.[1]

Before delving too deep into this discussion of Energy Medicine maybe it would be a good idea to set the stage with some elements of Quantum Physics.

Energy Medicine is discussed more in Chapter 3.

Quantum Physics and Mechanics

The sub atomic universe, the space between molecules was discovered when physicists started pushing the boundaries of known physics into new frontiers and looking deeper with more powerful microscopes and asking thought provoking questions.

The history of modern physics started in 1687 with Sir Isaac Newton publishing his theories on Gravity in a work entitled *Philosophiae Naturalis Principia Mathematica (Mathematical Principles of Natural Philosophy)* commonly known as the *Principia.*

> He calculated the force needed to hold the Moon in its orbit, as compared with the force pulling an object to the ground. He also calculated the centripetal force needed to hold a stone in a sling, and the relation between the length of a pendulum and the time of its swing. These early explorations were not soon exploited by Newton, though he studied astronomy and the problems of planetary motion.
>
> Correspondence with Hooke (1679-1680) redirected Newton to the problem of the path of a body subjected to a centrally directed force that varies as the inverse square of the distance; he determined it to be an ellipse, so informing Edmond Halley in August 1684. Halley's interest led Newton to demonstrate the relationship afresh, to compose a brief tract on mechanics, and finally to write the *Principia.*[2]

(Classical) Newtonian Physics has been taught in schools all around the world for about 300 years. This worldview sees matter being composed of atoms and molecules, protons and electrons – the big stuff.

Physicists on the other hand in the years since Newton, have increasingly been looking at the spaces in-between the atoms and molecules and have discovered that there is indeed a microcosm worth exploring.

Quantum Physics has been defined as the study of the behaviour of matter and energy at the molecular, atomic, nuclear and even smaller microscopic levels.

The founding fathers of Quantum physics most notably are: Max Planck, Niels Bohr, Werner Heisenberg, Erwin Schrödinger and Albert Einstein. Some of the others frequently mentioned are: Louis de Broglie, Max Born, John von Neumann, Paul Dirac, Wolfgang Pauli.

The Classical view of the world maintained that everything was influenced by cause and effect. Einstein's theory of Relativity reflected this worldview. He proposed that it was meaningless to speak of one body (molecule, individual, planet) moving and another body being still. Bodies can only be thought of as moving in relationship to each other; all motion is relative to some frame of reference, and the laws of nature apply unchanged, whatever that frame of reference.

In Einstein's mind it was impossible to reconcile the idea of waves turning into particles, as it was not in sync with the Theory of Relativity. So he focused his attentions elsewhere.

Some of his colleagues were proposing that while Relativity may be true at the molecular level and higher, on the microscopic quantum level these rules did not apply. Something else was happening, and so the concept of observers influencing waves of energy that in turn became particles ignited much controversy.

For instance: The theory of Non-Locality – Downward Causation.

The theory can be described like this:

A whole particle is split into two - particle A and B. Particle A is sent off in one direction and particle B going in the opposite direction, both end up being at the outer edges of the universe. If particle A is struck, particle B will instantly feel it.

Initially it looks like particle A was communicating with particle B faster than the speed of light. However, because of Einstein's theory of Relativity we know that nothing moves faster than the speed of light so something else must have communicated this information to particle B.

Niels Bohr and others suggested that the instant communication had something to do with both particles remembering that they were once interconnected prior to being split.

Particle A and B 'remembered' when they were a single undivided particle, this remembrance on the Quantum level is being part of the Unified Field. This field is also known as Holographic Universe or Living Matrix.

In essence this field emphasizes, "We are all One". From the cosmic dust speck hurtling through the Milky Way, to and including all the inhabitants of this Earth biosphere.

While Bohr realized that we were all connected his thoughts, theories and research could not provide the how. Another physicist, David Bohm, was able to provide an answer.

Bohm's book *Wholeness and the Implicate Order* (1983) gives a detailed explanation of implicate and explicate order of the universe.

There is a deeper level of reality the *implicate* (which means "enfolded") order, and our own level of existence is the *explicate*, or unfolded, order.[3]

Another explanation of this idea is: The material things we know so well are referred to as the 'explicate order'. In Bohmian terms; observable, measurable 'things' in the explicate order are entirely dependent upon the underlying relationships between things in the implicate order-for their very existence.[4]

Bohm believes that our almost universal tendency to fragment the world and ignore the dynamic interconnectedness of all this is responsible for many of our problems, not only in science but in our lives and our society as well.[5]

Quantum physicist John Hagelin was one of the many scientists who spoke in the movie "What the ?1$*! Bleep movie (2005).

[The] core basis of the Universe: we are all one. A single (self-aware) unified field of consciousness – non-material waves of vibration, information, and potential. Pure abstract potential existence, which rises in waves of vibration.

"Quantum is also a technical term, once known only to physicists but now growing in popular usage. The formal definition of quantum given by the eminent British physicist Stephen Hawking is 'the indivisible unit in which waves may be emitted or absorbed.'"[6]

This is how we can view Energy Medicine.

The macrocosm that is our body has a cellular memory of when we were that one-celled organism at the moment of conception. That one cell remembers when it was in fact two individual cells: part of our biological parents. This is on the molecular level.

On a deeper level the macrocosm of our individual self gets lost at the quantum level in the complexity of layers and in-between spaces that makes up who we are.

Connective fibres and tissues run and interact with the entire length of our bodies, which communicate with each other without the typical synaptic nerve - central nervous system relay.

Downward Causation or Non-locality is at work here.

This can help explain why one twin can feel the pain of the other who was injured. It is at this deep level that the cells of the twins are vibrating at the same frequency. There is no need to send silent waves of communication to one another, and distance is not a factor. How's that for instant messaging!

So what does this have to do with Energy Medicine practitioners?

When Energy practitioners are working with clients they are interacting with the subtle energies of the body, via the electromagnetic waves emitted from the practitioners hands. Or according to Candace Pert it could be the "free flow of information carried by the biochemicals of emotion, the neuropeptides and their receptors."[7]

The electromagnetic energy interacts with the subtle energies in the connective tissue. While the energy given may be at the client's head, the whole body is benefiting due to the electrical transmission provided by the connective tissue.

An experiment was done to test the concept of [an] energy exchange between a practitioner and client. The experimenters were able to prove by the use of an electrocardiogram (ECG) on one person and an electroencephalogram (EEG) on the other that there is indeed transference of energy from one to the other. It was also noted that on occasion a client would send energy to the practitioner.[8]

William Tiller has done his own research monitoring subtle energies from a healer and discovered some interesting information.

The information receivers (clairvoyants, etc.) and for ordinary subjects, no such pulses were observed. Instead of the usual 10-15 millivolt baseline with ~ 1 millivolt ripple, the ear lobe voltage often plunged −30 to −300 volts and then recovered to baseline in –0.5 to –10 seconds. This is an astoundingly large voltage pulse, -10^5 times normal! In a single 30 minute healing session that took place inside this special environment, one particular healer manifested 15 of these anomalously large voltage bursts (each greater than 30 volts) with each main burst being composed of 5-6 sub-pulses convolved in one envelope.[9]

It has also been noted that some practitioners may pick up or tune into the cellular trauma memories stored in their client's body. Somatic Recall is the name given to this response by biophysicist James Oschman.

Craniosacral practitioners have also experienced these events with their with clients however; they refer to Somatic Recall as "SomatoEmotional Release."[10]

Candace Pert quotes Craniosacral founder John Upledger to explain this event as "somato-emotional cysts, which are pockets of blocked emotion held in the body causing a breakdown in the energy flow and general health."[11]

Some physical therapists and massage therapists also report gleaning similar kinds of information from their clients.

As a side note not all practitioners experience this with every client, nor may they experience this each time they work on the same client.

The client on the other hand may remember the event in question at that moment or remember it days later. Or the client may not remember the event or trauma that the practitioner is picking up upon.

Gary Schwartz, PhD, and Linda Russek, PhD, Paul Pearsall, MD, have conducted research into the memories that are stored in heart muscle.

Heart transplantation is not simply a question of replacing an organ that no longer functions. The heart is often seen as source of love, emotions, and focus of personality traits. To gain insight into the problem of whether transplant patients themselves feel a change in personality after having received a donor heart, 47 patients who were transplanted over a period of 2 years in Vienna, Austria, were asked for an interview. Three groups of patients could be identified: 79% stated that their personality had not changed at all postoperatively. In this group, patients showed massive defense and denial reactions, mainly by rapidly changing the subject or making the question ridiculous. Fifteen per cent stated that their personality had indeed changed, but not because of the donor organ, but due to the life-threatening event. Six per cent (three patients) reported a distinct change of personality due to their new hearts. These incorporation fantasies forced them to change feelings and reactions and accept those of the donor. Verbatim statements of these heart transplant recipients show that there seem to be severe problems regarding graft incorporation, which are based on the age-old idea of the heart as a centre that houses feelings and forms the personality.[12]

Clearly this is only the tip of the iceberg regarding the ability of connective tissue or even muscle tissue being capable of storing memory. More research is definitely needed here.

In order for this cellular communication to happen the connective tissue needs to be hydrated. Proper hydration is vitally important for electrical impulse readings taken in science experiments - ECG readings and when working one-on-one with a client.

The amount of water is important as it takes 2 litres of water to replace, that which is lost during respiration each day. Never mind the amount of water needed for proper bowel and brain function. The blood is 80 percent water thus hydration levels are extremely important in blood chemistry.

Being suitably hydrated assists in the electrolyte (potassium, chloride, magnesium, calcium and sodium) balance that is vital for proper health. In order to avoid: muscle spasms, headaches, and irregular heart rhythms, etc.

In the absolute sense Modern Medicine has been using energy medicine for years just in a different form. Any time a patient is hooked up to a monitor or is asked to have a scan of some kind this is energy medicine.

> Modern researchers have developed the magnetic biopsy, the electrical biopsy, and the optical biopsy. Transcutaneous nerve stimulators, cardiac pacemakers and defibrillators, lasers, electrocautery, and pulsing magnetic field therapy are examples of energy treatment modalities that are part of conventional medicine. Controversial or not, energy medicine based on the use of medical equipment is alive and well in hospitals, clinics, and medical research centers.[13]

The fields of electrical or magnetic energy of that patient are being measured, to see if they are functioning within an optimum range.

If this optimal range is not present then a process begins to determine what is going on or what needs to be done in order to restore the human body to a healthier condition.

Chapter Review:

Everything in our known universe is composed of vibrations. Our invisible world is made up of particles, atoms and sub-atomic elements that move and vibrate, change shape and influence their neighbours. It is these subtle energy vibrations that an Energy Medicine practitioner connects with when doing their work, stimulating the body to repair it – helping the body restore homeostasis.

Chapter 2

The Mechanical Human – Not!

Medicine has been part of all cultures whether the indigenous people of the Americas, the Aborigines of Australia, the Ancient Egyptians, Sumerians or inhabitants of the Indus Valley. The roots of modern medicine go back to the early Greek and Italian nature-philosophers, who viewed health within the context of being a priest, connected to local temples offering prayers, studying the elements of nature – herbs, wind, fire and water and communing with oracles.

Then came Classical Greek philosophers Hippocrates, Aristotle, Socrates who used logic and reason to discern the cause of illness.

The theory of the Four Humours: heat and cold, moisture and dryness and the delicate balance they must maintain for us to be healthy. At this time there was also the occasional foray into the body itself to understand the workings of the heart and blood vessels. However, for the most part the body was left intact, as it was viewed as sacred. This view was maintained until well into the late Renaissance.

The Renaissance began in Northern Italy during the fourteenth century, and travelled to Northern and Western Europe by the migration of some of its more forward thinkers.

The shackles of insecurity created by the fall of Rome and the Northern invaders, fell away to expose a European mind thirsty for knowledge.

Prior to the Renaissance, the Church was the only constant in a person's life. The church was a place of solace for the weak and weary. It was the place where a young man from a noble family could get an education. If you were sick the hospital infirmary dressed your body in poultices and unguents then administered the last rites to assist the passage of your soul.

While the Church may have had its bad moments, on the whole it was the glue that held a community together.

With the advent of the Renaissance, men were no longer willing to be schooled only by the Church. A yearning for more stimulated a quest for knowledge from an earlier age.

This led to a revival in Greek and Roman classical literature, art and philosophy. It was with this backdrop that numerous investigations of natural events, the movement of the heavens and the development of modern interests and ideals were created.

The Church did not normally discuss these things. The Church's task was to take care of your mortal soul. They made sure that you confessed your sins so when the end came you too could sit with the Heavenly host.

RENÉ DESCARTES (1596-1650) was one of these Renaissance men. His famous quotation "Cogito Ergo Sum" ("I think, therefore I am.") pretty much sums up the next 400 years.

But the most important contribution Descartes made was his philosophical writings. Descartes, who was convinced that science and mathematics could be used to explain everything in nature, was the first to describe the physical universe in terms of matter and motion, seeing the universe as a giant mathematically designed engine. Descartes wrote three important texts: Discourse on the Method of Rightly Conducting the Reason and Seeking Truth in the Sciences, Meditations on First Philosophy, and Principles of Philosophy.

With this discussion the Church felt it necessary to establish certain boundaries regarding this enquiry. Items of a religious nature and theology were to remain the domain of the Church.

Descartes separated church and science; these things were now compartmentalized. Medical science = medical practice and science. He argued with the church that this model would not threaten the authority of the church and in no way did it threaten theology.

The view of man being created by God was still viable, however the body was poked, prodded and dissected in order to understand what was really happening beneath the surface of the skin.

This compartmentalization by Descartes equated man to a machine; we are the sum of our parts.

Small realizations about the human body were replaced by bigger realizations. These inquiries lead to trying to understand the living world around us. By seeing life as a logical progression from small one-celled organisms and so on to its termination as humans was a comforting feeling to those who felt that Science was the new Church.

The human has become a microcosm, a stand-alone feature, which replaces the macrocosmic human view as being a component of nature. We are our own universe, with the world dancing to our whims; we are separate and distinct from everything else.

This need to classify everything and seeing things broken down into its component parts is like a two year old learning its mother tongue. Pointing at everything they see in order to know what they are — bus, car, shoe, cat, dog, bird, tree, cookie.

Science did the same objectifying things into lists, the classification of plants (flora) and animals (fauna) into the Linnaeus taxonomic nomenclature of domain, kingdom, phylum, class, order, family, genus, species.

Then science itself was categorised: Biology: the study of life, Astronomy the scientific study of celestial objects, Geology the study of the earth, Oceanography the study of oceans, Chemistry the study of elements and the list goes on.

We are Reductionists, compartmentalizing life and becoming specialists to the Nth degree, no longer do we see the forest because we only see one element of one tree – a microcosm.

Physicians have been chastised for this "ideology of "reductionism" – when it is taken to mean seeing illness, at least in principle, in terms of physical or biochemical changes alone (associated with laboratory investigations and medical technology).[1]

"The focus of most contemporary medicine has been more on disease detection, diagnosis, and treatment, and only very recently on health promotion and disease prevention."[2]

To their credit Ecologists who study the relationship of organisms to each other and to their physical surroundings. They study the macrocosm, and if we are discussing human ecology this is vitally important to us as a species. In some respects I would have to say we have lost sight of the context of interrelationship.

The current world condition called global warming is not just a condition affecting only those who live in the Polar Regions and where glaciers are. This situation is affecting all of Earth's inhabitants equally: polar, temperate, sub-tropical and tropical. It is affecting land, sea, air and the ozone. If we ever needed an indication that our lives are part of the web of life – this is it.

This is "old-paradigm thinking, which views each of us as an isolated entity, separated from others and from our environment, living apart from the whole and not connected to it."[3]

What industrialized countries or we the G 8 and G 20 countries do affects and impacts the technologically challenged or Third World countries who also live on this planet.

These technologically challenged countries are struggling to ensure all aspects of their culture, flora and fauna and natural resources are kept intact. To be sure this is no easy task, but what does this really mean.

We need to pull back from our microscopes and look at the big picture, the Holistic view.

"Nowadays, holism is also commonly viewed as summarizing

the "modern" definition of health stemming from the World Health Organization. This sees health as a state of complete physical, mental and social well-being, and not merely the absence of physical illness. (wellness)..."[4]

True health is more than just the absence of disease.

Each individual (plant or animal) is a fully vibrant being, interacting with, responding to and respecting their environment. This environment is inclusive encompassing all things that move on land, swim in oceans, and breathe the air, as we are all connected to this biosphere.

The Holistic Approach

Holism
Traditional – focused on the whole
Functioning
Integration
Web of relationship
System approach
Wellness
Inclusive – value all
Watchful waiting
Minimal intervention
Understanding
Enhancement

The Conventional Approach

Reductionism
Conventional – focused on parts
Mechanics
Isolation
Divorced from context
Specialized medicine

Pathology
Separation – scepticism
Aggressive intervention leading to heroic measures
Knowledge
Fixing

Traditional healers, the medicine men and women around the world know the Holistic view and see the world this context. They are at one or in harmony with their environment: land, water, animals, the seen and the unseen.

In the past, modern society has ridiculed these Traditional healers as being backward and superstitious. Science is just starting to validate what these men and women have practiced for centuries.

Herbal almanacs are no longer anecdotal and mere folklore.

Rainforests are a vital source of medicines. Today, less than 1% of the world's tropical forest plants have been tested for pharmaceutical properties, yet at least 25% of all modern drugs came originally from rainforests. Most were first discovered and used by indigenous peoples.

Annual worldwide sales of plant-derived pharmaceuticals currently total $20 billion. These include such drugs as Digitoxin, Vincristine, Emetine, Physostigamine, Atropine, Morphine, Resepine, D-Tubocurarine, and Quinine. All were first used by rainforest shamans and healers.

An impressive 70% of all plants known to have anti-tumour properties come from tropical rainforests. Any one of these could lead to breakthroughs in the treatment of cancer. The potential of this living pharmaceutical factory remains almost completely untapped.[5]

The potential and fragility of the rainforests as an invaluable source of medicine is clearly illustrated in the following account from the World Rainforest Report no. 26. Oct 1992, Rainforest Information Centre, Lismore, Australia

> Starting with twigs from a Malaysian gum tree, researchers in 1991 isolated a compound that blocked the spread of the AIDS virus in human cells. The team sent biologists racing back to Malaysia for more samples from the tree. But when they got to the swamp, the tree was gone, it had been cut down. And no tree found since has produced the same compound." No identical trees have been found in the immediate area and samples from the same species found elsewhere did not yield the same compound.

> In Sarawak, the Penan people use over 50 medicinal plants which they harvest from the primary forest – plants that are used as poison antidotes, contraceptives, clotting agents, general tonics, stimulants, disinfectants, remedies for headaches, fever, cuts and bruises, boils, snake bite, toothache, diarrhoea, skin infections and rashes, and for setting bones.[6]

In First Nations culture it is well known that a person only takes what they need as we are only borrowing it from our children's children. Conserving is not only for the future seven generations, but back seven generations too.

When viewing our client from a Holistic point of view everything is important.

If they are sick, what were the stages (symptoms) that the body went through to get to this stage?

This is a key reference point in **Homeopathy**. If a client had a sore throat there are 6 possible remedies to take. But it all depends on the symptoms:

Front of mouth normal, back of throat yellowish and coated, person craves fresh air, tonsil abscess threatening.

This client would receive Calcarea sulph. 6c[7]

Note: this **an example only** not medical advice, please seek assistance from a licensed health practitioner.

This is part of the TCM Theory and Diagnostics II course offered by the Toronto School of **Traditional Chinese Medicine**.

The four basic diagnostic methods are:

1) Inquiring about a patient's current and past medical history, collecting detailed information about the cause, symptoms and development, as well as diagnosis and treatment of diseases;
2) Palpation of the body and the pulse;
3) Inspection of the tongue and the general appearance; and
4) Auscultation and olfaction.[8]

Modern pharmacology often strives to isolate and administer the active ingredients of a substance such as herbs. In TCM the entire, unprocessed substance is most often used, with the belief that different parts of the herb interact with each other, actually enhancing the 'active' ingredient in the herb while at the same time neutralizing potential side effects by keeping the substance intact.[9]

Ayurveda is a system of traditional medicine native to India.

At the Ayurvedic Institute in Albuquerque, New Mexico they teach students about herbs, nutrition, panchakarma cleansing, acupressure massage, Yoga and Sanskrit.

It has been said that in Ayurvedic medicine illness has 6 stages (one being minor and 6 being terminal) of pathogenesis, (disease diagnosis) in modern medicine they appear to only focus on the last one stage 6, which is the stage of no hope or a cure.

As you can see these are just a few examples of what is offered by other inclusive health care systems. Here it is possible to get a picture of the client's web of life, and discover what are all the important pieces that make up the whole.

The Traditional approach to health care is proactive, holistic and looks at prevention as a way to keep their clients healthy. The focus is on Wellness with a personal touch. Clients are educated and empowered.

The Conventional approach to health care is reactive, reductionist and disease oriented. The focus is on the compartmentalized parts and technological tools. It has been noted some medical personnel miss having that more intimate contact with their patients.

It is well known that death by drug interactions and side effects have been worked into the statistical efficacy and profitability of most pharmaceutical drugs.

The consumer, our clients and patients are initiating changes in modern medicine.

The Integrative Medicine approach is taking the best of both worlds.

The client is an integral part of this new model. By feeling listened to, respected and empowered the client is more inclined to comply with a treatment plan worked out with the health care provider.

Complementary and Alternative Medicine (CAM) is often not accepted because it is culturally different, because mechanisms are not clearly understood or are explained in a way that is contrary to our belief system or currently accepted medical and scientific concepts. Modern medicine requires an understanding that fits its current constructs. CAM challenges these paradigms, and perhaps will facilitate a paradigm shift. This shift will only occur when data is unequivocal, hence the need for well-designed, repeatable trials to determine what does and does not work. CAM must be willing to undergo this study and to stand up to scientific scrutiny.[10]

In the United States some new doctors take the modern version of the Hippocratic oath created by Louis Lasagna in 1964. By incorporating an Integrative approach to medicine this excerpted phrase may carry more weight. "I will apply, for the benefit of the sick, all measures [that] are required, avoiding those twin traps of over treatment and therapeutic nihilism."[11]

Mind-Body Connection

Could this possibly be why we think of our bodies as machines?

Once this automaton is turned on at birth, it functions pretty much on autopilot until it breaks down. Then there is a mad dash scramble to return this body back to normal; or the re-establishment of autopilot.

We are not just our bodies, minds, blood, and various physical systems. Nor are we just composed of atoms and molecules that function according to the laws of physics and chemistry.

Our body relays vital bits of information the length and breadth of itself every moment. Levels of hunger, thirst, pain, immune function, alkaline-acid balance, electrolyte balance and etc. All of this happens by itself, it happens without your conscious awareness.

In the book Quantum Healing, Dr. Deepak Chopra shares a related thought.

[It] is my belief that consciousness creates reality... that expectation decisively influences outcome ... and that awareness, attention, and intention should be as much a part of health care as drugs, radiation, and surgery.[12]

The most exciting property of the living matrix (our body) is the ability of the entire network to generate and conduct vibrations. In this way, every part is informed of what all other parts are doing.[13]

This communication can be in a myriad of ways: the electrical conductivity of nerves, chemical signalling hormones, chromosomal replication by our DNA and emotions.

Science is becoming keenly aware the role our emotions play in our lives. Our emotions are more than the primal urges to find food, have shelter and procreate. Emotions give colour to our world: joy, sorrow, anger, contentment, love and hate. We are discovering that emotions can also be friend or foe.

Emotions are constantly regulating what we experience as 'reality.' The decision about what sensory information travels to your brain and what gets filtered out depends on what signals the receptors are receiving from the peptides[1].[14]

"Emotional states or moods are produced by the various neuropeptide[2] ligands[3], and what we experience as an emotion or a feeling is also a mechanism for activating a particular neuronal circuit – *simultaneously throughout the brain and body* – which generates a behavior involving the whole creature, with all the necessary physiological changes that behavior would require."[15]

The phrase "sticks and stones my break my bones but names can never hurt me", could not be further from the truth. Harmful and hurtful words can indeed cause pain; they can even challenge our concept of self. If we have a negative self-image it can lead to depression, psychological blocks, emotional eating or purging, self-loathing, self-mutilation or worse death.

If we do have a negative self-image, we may have the mindset that nothing we do is ever good enough; it will never work so why bother. In effect we will sabotage anything and everything because we don't believe we are worth it. So we find excuses not to start that exercise program to shed that couple of extra pounds we have gained over the recent cold winter. Or we put off tackling a task in the job jar because it will take too long, and I don't have the time, tools or whatever to get it done. I am sure we all know someone we could relate this to; it could even be ourselves.

Instead of looking at and focusing on these could haves and other excuses, a better use of our time would be to focus on the following. I love myself enough to get this job done, or I love myself enough to want to embrace a vibrant healthy lifestyle.

Get rid of the shoulds and shouldn'ts and consequent feelings of guilt because they only keep you in victim mode – poor me – and you stay mired in the cesspool of your own pity party.

How many of you were told it is better to give than to receive? I know I was, and it has taken me a long time to allow myself to receive compliments, gifts and other things and feel comfortable about it.

Some of us are not very comfortable or good at doing nothing. We are so used to being humans doing (having to be productive) we have forgotten to be a human be-ing. Or maybe it has something to do with hearing 'idle hands are the devil's tools; workshop; playthings or handiwork'. You may have your own version of this saying.

I am not suggesting that we become narcissists, however I would like to suggest that we treat ourselves with more compassion and kindness. It may be time to be a little more selfish.

Take the time to do good things for "us" like meditation; whatever it is it doesn't have to provide you with a certificate, diploma, or degree. Go run in the sprinkler with the kids or grandkids if you have them, it would be good for your soul.

Speaking of meditation, it is an excellent way to re-establish the mind-body connection.

Anna Wise has written a lovely book for those who wish to use their brains more effectively.

The back cover of the book states '... how brain waves influence mental states and how to use this knowledge to heighten mental acuity and awareness.'[16]

The book has exercises in print form and they are also on CD to assist you in providing an optimal experience.

There are four types of brain wave patterns listed Beta, Alpha, Delta and Theta.

Beta brain waves are the fastest, (13-30 Hz) most common brain-wave pattern for a waking state of consciousness. They are produced by your thinking mind – your conscious thought process. Beta is what you use to navigate and negotiate through your everyday life. Your beta can encompass high anxiety and panic – the list-making, judging, critiquing, and continual commenting that can be present in an over –active mind – as well as creative, clear, alert, attentive thinking.

...beta is vital to the creative process and assists in its expression.

Alpha brain waves are the next fastest (8-12 Hz) frequencies. Alpha is our relaxed detached awareness, or daydreaming mind. It provides the lucidity and vividness of our imagery.

Alpha's primary and indispensable importance is that it is the bridge or link between the conscious and the subconscious mind. It helps you to remember your dreams upon awakening and keeps you in touch with your deep inner meditation world.

Theta brain waves (4-8 Hz) are produced by the subconscious mind. They are present in dreaming sleep and the REM (rapid eye movement) state. The subconscious holds our long-term memory and is also the storehouse of creative inspiration and the repository of suppressed creativity, as well as repressed psychological material. This is where we hold our "stuff" or "baggage" – the unclear emotional material.

It is through theta that we make our strongest spiritual connection. This is also the place where we get those "ah-ha" experiences.

For those of us in the holistic field this is where we want our clients to be in order to heal their body or mind, theta is the place where the healing most readily enters your being and makes a deep, penetrating impact.

Delta (less than 4 Hz) is the lowest and slowest of all frequencies - the unconscious mind. Delta is still present when all of the other frequencies turn off in sleep, giving you deep restorative rest. In some people, delta is present in a waking state in combination with other brain waves. As such, it acts as a kind of "radar" or unconscious scanning device that underlies our intuition, our empathy, and our instinctual action. It also offers that true sense of inner knowing that provides deep levels of psychic awareness.

Delta waves are often evident in people in the helping professions – people who need to reach out and enter into someone else's mental, psychological, or emotional being. Delta can also be present in large quantities in hands-on healers and in those who are "people people".

...it's a very primal and animalistic brain wave. Delta waves allow you to glean information that isn't available on a conscious level. From the negative point of view, delta can also be used for hypervigilance.

Delta has also been connected with the concept of the collective unconscious.[17]

Throughout the book Quantum Healing, Dr.Chopra explores the use of Ayurvedic medicine to heal the body. This form of whole body healing strongly believes in the power of meditation.

Science had been looking at the scientific side of meditation, trying to figure out exactly what it does. It appears that it can "in fact induce profound change, far beyond the simple relaxation that most people use it for in the West, even beyond the medical applications of relieving stress, reducing blood pressure, and so on."[18]

Dr. Chopra also feels that by being able to access deep levels of mediation we can alter the "hidden blueprint of intelligence"[19] this involves our DNA, the mechanism which talks – chemically speaking – to the body-mind.

At these "deeper states were experienced as absolute inner silence, a feeling of vast expansion, and a profound knowingness. The mind was emptied of all specific thoughts but left with the clear awareness of 'I know everything'."[20]

As you can see by accessing these various meditative states they will help us in all aspects of our life, so we can be focused when needed and more fully relaxed during downtime.

Living in the Modern World

If you were to sit down at the end of the day and take stock, do you feel that you are further ahead of your parents or behind?

I ask this question because social scientists have said that this generation (current child-bearing adults) will strive to make their offspring's lives better than their own.

Depending on who you ask, the answer might range from yes, it is greatly improved to no, not really. The not really better folks are the ones who feel like a hamster running the wheel in its cage, or like a dog chasing its tail.

This endless game of catch-up is not healthy, neither mentally nor physically. Some of us hate our lives and wonder how do we get off this merry-go-round. The dreams from our childhood have vanished and we are stuck in the 9 to 5 drudgery of a working world. With the constant question being "exactly how many days are left until my vacation."

With this rather depressing scenario what is there to feel joyful about?

What does this do to stress levels?

What does this do to relationships with loved ones, extended family and friends?

Who has time or the energy at the end of the day or week to do much more than vegetate on the couch?

Who has time to cook any more, processed foods are so much easier for a family on the run.

Enough already!

This type of frenetic activity is going to kill us and it already is.

We desperately need to restore some balance in all areas of our lives - work, sleep, health, play, and quiet time.

But our new understanding of neuropeptides and receptors has enabled us to see more of what is going on in conditions of stress. When stress prevents the molecules of emotion from flowing freely where needed, the largely autonomic processes that are regulated by peptide flow, such as breathing, blood flow, immunity, digestion, and elimination, collapse down to a few simple feedback loops and upset the normal healing response.[21]

If we revisit the aspects of a Holistic approach, the focus is on:

- wholeness
- robust health
- vibrant
- an integral part in the web of life

Life in general needs to slow down. Have you heard that "slow " food instead of "fast" food is catching on?

Savor the moments in life, there will be less stress, better digestion of your food, less rage, and a whole lot more compassion to be shared with others.

Get out and smell the roses, go for a walk, watch the sunset, gaze at the stars.

Stop letting the tail [our frenetic lives] wag the dog.

Trust me, your body will thank you for it.

Maybe it is time to follow Candace Pert's lead and think of disease-related stress in the following way, "in terms of information overload, a condition in which the mind-body network is so taxed by unprocessed sensory input in the form of suppressed trauma or undigested emotions that it has become bogged down and cannot flow freely, sometimes even working against itself, at cross-purposes."[22]

During a Wellness Conference in Milwaukee, Candace Pert and Dr. Brian Luke Seaward and a few others were answering questions regarding mind-body health.

Candace: The discussion so far has left out bodywork: the touch therapies of massage, chiropractic, and any other modality that includes the body as a means of healing the mind and emotions. It's true, we do store some memory in the brain, but by far, the deeper, older messages are stored in the body and must be accessed through the body. Your body is your subconscious mind, and you can't heal it by talk alone.

Brian Seaward adds: "The body becomes the battlefield for the war games of the mind. All the unresolved thoughts and emotions, the negativity we hold on to, shows up in the body and makes us sick."[23]

As you can see an injury whether mental, emotional or physical that affects one organ or limb of our bodies can deeply impact the rest of the self.

If you truly love yourself and want to have the best of what life can give you make the change because you're worth it!

Chapter Review

To quote an old television by-line – "You've come a long way baby!"

Yes, we have, in effect we have come full circle.

Initially, as hunter-gatherers we were in tune with the cycles of nature and co-existed with our environments.

Over time we have forgotten or started to think of ourselves as superior to nature and its inhabitants.

With the wisdom of years we are remembering and rediscovering that our actions impact those around us and everything else that lives with us.

This wisdom is also carries over to how humans view their own bodies; no longer is it "the knee bone is connected to the hipbone". Now we are investing in the whole person, mentally, emotionally, physically and spiritually. We are then extrapolating the health of this person to the health of his or her environment: within the home, outside the home – the community, and the extending it to our global village.

Chapter 3

How Governments view Complementary and Alternative Therapies

Initially, a small portion of the public became disenchanted with conventional medicine, and was drawn to exploring alternative forms of healing.

At first, the name Alternative was a good adjective to describe the service provided by persons not working in the current medical model. Now, as the public is becoming more familiar with the various healing modalities, the term Complementary seems more appropriate.

For those of us in the Complementary field this has been a welcome change as we recognize the importance of conventional health care providers. As we move to Integrative Medicine, we would like to be seen as partners, part of the health care team that works with clients (patients) to assist them in achieving optimal health.

Like all new things this road has been fraught with bumps and potholes. One way to assist the public in understanding the range of modalities listed under Complementary health is to educate everyone.

In Canada we are relying heavily upon the work done in the United States by the National Center for Complementary and Alternative Medicine (NCCAM) at the National Institute of Health (NIH).

http://nccam.nih.gov/health/whatiscam/energy/energymed.htm

The current NCCAM definition is an easy to read eight-page article located at www.nccam.nih.gov

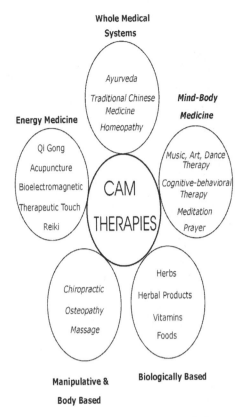

Here are some of the highlights. Some of the more important pieces have been cut and pasted into this chapter but the author encourages you to visit the above website.

Energy medicine is a domain in [Complementary and Alternative Medicine] CAM that deals with energy fields of two types:[1]

Veritable, which can be measured
Putative, which have yet to be measured

The **veritable** energies employ mechanical vibrations (such as sound) and electromagnetic forces, including visible light, magnetism, monochromatic radiation (such as laser beams), and rays from other parts of the electromagnetic spectrum. They involve the use of specific, measurable wavelengths and frequencies to treat patients.

In contrast, **putative** energy fields (also called biofields) have defied measurement to date by reproducible methods. Therapies involving putative energy fields are based on the concept that human beings are infused with a subtle form of energy. This vital energy or life force is known under different names in different cultures, such as qi in traditional Chinese medicine, the vital energy or life force proposed to regulate a person's spiritual, emotional, mental, and physical health and to be influenced by the opposing forces of yin and yang. In traditional Chinese medicine: a whole medical system that originated in China.

Examples of practices involving putative energy fields include:

Reiki and Johrei, both of Japanese origin

Qi gong, a Chinese practice

Healing touch, in which the therapist is purported to identify imbalances and correct a client's energy by passing his or her hands over the patient

Intercessory prayer, in which a person intercedes through prayer on behalf of another

(cut)

Scope of the Research

Veritable Energy Medicine

There are many well-established uses for the application of measurable energy fields to diagnose or treat diseases: electro-magnetic fields in magnetic resonance imaging, cardiac pacemakers, radiation therapy, ultraviolet light for psoriasis, laser keratoplasty, and more. There are many other claimed uses as well. (cut)

For example, both static and pulsating electromagnetic

therapies have been employed.

Magnetic Therapy

Static magnets have been used for centuries in efforts to relieve pain or to obtain other alleged benefits (e.g., increased energy). Numerous anecdotal reports have indicated that individuals have experienced significant, and at times dramatic, relief of pain after the application of static magnets over a painful area. Although the literature on the biological effects of magnetic fields is growing, there is a paucity of data from well-structured, clinically sound studies. However, there is growing evidence that magnetic fields can influence physiological processes.

Millimeter Wave Therapy

Low-power millimeter wave (MW) irradiation elicits biological effects, and clinicians in Russia and other parts of Eastern Europe have used it in past decades to treat a variety of conditions, ranging from skin diseases and wound healing to various types of cancer, gastrointestinal and cardiovascular diseases, and psychiatric illnesses.

Sound Energy Therapy

Sound energy therapy, sometimes referred to as vibrational or frequency therapy, includes music therapy as well as wind chime and tuning fork therapy. The presumptive basis of its effect is that specific sound frequencies resonate with specific organs of the body to heal and support the body.

Light Therapy

Light therapy is the use of natural or artificial light to treat various ailments, but unproven uses of light extend to lasers, colors, and monochromatic lights. High-intensity light therapy - the use of natural or artificial light — including colored light and high-intensity light — for health purposes.

Energy Medicine Involving Putative Energy Fields

The concept that sickness and disease arise from imbalances in the vital energy field of the body has led to many forms of therapy. In TCM, a series of approaches are taken to rectify the flow of qi, such as herbal medicine, acupuncture (and its various versions), qi gong, diet, and behavior changes.

Acupuncture

Of these approaches, acupuncture is the most prominent therapy to promote qi flow along the meridians.

Qi Gong

Qi gong, another energy modality that purportedly can restore health, is practiced widely in the clinics and hospitals of China.

Whole Medical Systems and Energy Medicine

Although modalities such as acupuncture and qi gong have been studied separately; TCM uses combinations of treatments (e.g., herbs, acupuncture, and qi gong) in practice. Similarly, Ayurvedic medicine uses combinations of herbal medicine, yoga, and meditation. . (For more information on TCM and Ayurvedic medicine, see NCCAM's backgrounder "Whole Medical Systems: An Overview.")

Homeopathy

One Western approach with implications for energy medicine is homeopathy: a whole medical system that originated in Europe. Homeopathy seeks to stimulate the body's ability to heal itself by giving very small doses of highly diluted substances that in larger doses would produce illness or symptoms (an approach called "like cures like").

Therapeutic Touch and Related Practices

Numerous other practices have evolved over the years to

promote or maintain the balance of vital energy fields in the body. Examples of these modalities include Therapeutic Touch: a therapy in which practitioners pass their hands over another person's body with the intent to use their own perceived healing energy to identify energy imbalances and promote health, healing touch, Reiki, Johrei, vortex healing, and polarity therapy.

Distant Healing

Proponents of energy field therapies also claim that some of these therapies can act across long distances. For example, the long-distance effects of external qi gong have been studied in China and summarized in the book Scientific Qigong Exploration, which has been translated into English.

Physical Properties of Putative Energy Fields

There has always been an interest in detecting and describing the physical properties of putative energy fields. Kirlian photography, aura imaging, and gas discharge visualization are approaches for which dramatic and unique differences before and after therapeutic energy attunements or treatments have been claimed.

The United Kingdom has been wrestling with definitions regarding the Complementary and Alternative Medicine also.[2]

The House of Lords report classified complementary and alternative therapies into three groups and related many of its recommendations to this classification.

Categories of complementary and alternative therapies

Group 1: Professionally organized alternative therapies

Acupuncture
Chiropractic

Herbal medicine
Homoeopathy
Osteopathy

Group 2: Complementary therapies

Alexander technique
Aromatherapy
Bach and other flower extracts
Bodywork therapies, including massage
Counselling stress therapy
Hypnotherapy
Meditation
Reflexology
Shiatsu
Healing
Maharishi Ayurvedic medicine
Nutritional medicine
Yoga

Group 3: Alternative disciplines

3a: Long established and traditional systems of healthcare
Anthroposophical medicine
Ayurvedic medicine
Chinese herbal medicine
Eastern medicine (Tibb)
Naturopathy
Traditional Chinese medicine
3b: Other alternative disciplines
Crystal therapy
Dowsing
Iridology
Kinesiology

Radionics

As more research is done in these fields the categories may change not only within each country but also globally.

The World Health Organization that is part of the United Nations published in its bulletin a review by Charlie Changli Xue on the following: Volume 86, Number 1, January 2008, 1-80.

Traditional, complementary and alternative medicine: policy and public health perspectives[3]

Traditional medicine is an amorphous concept that comprises a range of long-standing and still evolving practices based on diverse beliefs and theories. Bodeker and Burford point out the dichotomous situation of particular forms of traditional medicine being practised in their countries of origin and also in countries to which they have been "imported". They suggest that the term "traditional, complementary and alternative medicine" (TCAM) is a more appropriate term to describe such traditional therapies globally.

Health care can broadly be divided into modern (conventional, orthodox, Western or allopathic) and traditional (indigenous, complementary, alternative or integrative). The former is clearly defined, with minor regional variations in its underlying philosophy and clinical methods. In modern medicine, knowledge expansion is achieved through scientific research, which can involve global collaboration and commitment. Such research is well supported financially by industry, governments and philanthropic organizations. This is in sharp contrast to the situation with TCAM.[4]

When the buying public wants to build a deck in their back yard, get their roof repaired, or buy a new car, nine times out of ten they are required to do a little legwork. They talk to friends they trust and see what companies or services they are happy with. If friends can't help then off to the classified section of the phone book, (paper or internet) and call some of the numbers listed for a quote.

Depending on the nature of the job, you may ask for referrals to see if the business does a good job, at a fair price and will stand by the work they do.

The same can be applied to any practitioner in the Complementary health field. Our clients want to know that the health practitioner is fully trained, knowledgeable and professional.

This equates to displaying your qualifications on the wall, continuing to educate yourself about what is new in your field and join a professional organization that applies to your field.

If this professional organization does a newsletter see if you can write an article. This can add credibility to your name. Doing research in your field will add credibility to both of you.

Research Design

The mechanics required to design a scientific research paper are beyond the scope of this book. Suffice it to say, depending on your field of inquiry you may need to speak with a statistician, scientist and or medical person at a college, university or research facility.

In Canada we have The Canadian Interdisciplinary Network for CAM Research (IN-CAM), which was officially launched in January 2004. Their mission is to foster a sustainable, well-connected, highly trained Complementary and Alternative Medicine (CAM) research community in Canada that is internationally recognized and known for both its excellence in research and its contributions to understanding CAM and its use.[5]

The United States also has many agencies researching Complementary and Alternative Medicine. In addition to NCCAM there is Agency for Healthcare Research and Quality. http://www.ahrq.gov/

The International Society for Complementary Medicine Research (ISCMR) is a worldwide not-for-profit professional association devoted to fostering co-operative and multidisciplinary research and development as well as the application of knowledge in the fields of Complementary, Traditional and Integrated Medicine. http://www.iscmr.org/

In general terms the current Gold standard in medical research is the Double blind, randomized double control trial. Some studies have a triple control, if you choose to do this it would depend on the nature of the research design.

IN-CAM has a section on its website which describes research methods.

The first item on IN-CAM's website is a link to the NCCAM website and an introduction to clinical trials.

As the time of writing the link is broken, the search engine at the NCCAM website provided an active link. http://nccam.nih .gov/research/clinicaltrials/factsheet/

This is a definition from the NCCAM clinical trials website:

3. What is a clinical trial?

A clinical trial is a research study in which a treatment or therapy is tested in people to see whether it is safe and effective. The information learned from clinical trials helps to improve health care and to keep people healthier. Researchers also conduct clinical trials to find out which treatments are more effective than others. The results from trials can also contribute to our understanding of diseases and conditions—for example, how a disease progresses or how it affects different systems in the body.

Clinical trials are also called medical research, research studies, or clinical studies. Each trial follows a protocol—a written, detailed plan that explains why there is a need for the study, what it is intended to do, and how it will be conducted. The protocol is written by the trial's principal investigator (the person who is in charge of the trial).

4. What are the major types of clinical trials?

Clinical trials are used to study many aspects of medical care:

- Treatment trials test treatments for a specific disease or condition.
- Supportive care trials, also called quality of life trials, study ways of making sick people more comfortable and giving them a better quality of life.
- Prevention trials study ways to reduce the chance that people who are healthy, but may be at risk for a disease, will develop the disease.
- Early detection or screening trials study new ways of finding diseases or conditions in people who are at risk, before they have any signs or symptoms.
- Diagnostic trials test new ways to identify, more accurately and earlier, whether people have diseases and conditions.

Clinical trials have sometimes been thought of as a last resort for those who have a disease and have tried all other treatment options. This is not true. There are trials for healthy people

NCCAM-3

(for example, to study disease prevention) and trials for all different types and stages of diseases.

5. What are the different phases of a clinical trial?

Because the therapy will be tested in people, before a clinical trial can start, there needs to be some evidence that it is likely to work. This evidence can come either from previous research studies in animals or from reported information on its use by people.

Clinical trials take place in phases. In each phase, different research questions are answered.

The following are types of questions that each phase helps to answer:

- Phase I: What is the safe dose? How does the treatment affect the human body? How should the treatment be given?
- Phase II: Does the therapy treat the disease or cure the condition?
- Phase III: Is the treatment better than, the same as, or worse than the standard (or most widely accepted) treatment? If there is no standard treatment available, is it better than, the same as, or worse than a placebo? (Placebos are explained below.)

6. What are some common elements of clinical trials?

Trials can be randomized. Each participant in a randomized trial is assigned by chance (through a computer or a table of random numbers) to one of two groups:

- The investigational group, made up of people who will receive the therapy, also called the active treatment
- The control group, made up of people who will receive either the standard treatment (if there is one) for their disease or condition, or a placebo

Each participant has an equal chance of being assigned to either group. In some complex trials, there are more than two groups. Randomization is used in all phase III studies and in some phase II studies. It gives the best chance of knowing that the study results are caused by the treatment and not some other factor, such as people's choices or beliefs.

Trials can be double-blind. This means that neither the researchers nor the participants know who has been assigned to which group. Blinding is another way to help minimize the chance of bias influencing the trial results. The information is kept on file at a central office, so if there is an urgent need for the research team to find out who was assigned the active treatment, they can.

Researchers design clinical trials to have one or more

endpoints. An endpoint is a measure that determines whether the treatment under study has an effect. An example of an endpoint is whether a person's tumor shrinks after receiving chemotherapy.

NCCAM-4

7. What is a placebo?

A placebo is designed to resemble as much as possible the treatment being studied in a clinical trial, except that the placebo is inactive. An example of a placebo is a pill containing sugar instead of the drug being studied. By giving one group of participants a placebo and the other group the active treatment, the researchers can compare how the two groups respond and get a truer picture of the active treatment's effects.

Another type of placebo is called a "sham" procedure. When the treatment under study is a procedure (not a drug or other substance), a sham procedure may be designed that resembles the active treatment but does not have any active treatment qualities. For example, in a clinical trial of acupuncture, the sham procedure might consist of placing acupuncture needles in areas of the body that are not expected (from previous knowledge) to have any therapeutic response.

In recent years, the definition of placebo has been expanded to include other things that could have an effect on the results of health care. Examples include how a patient and a health care provider interact, how a patient feels about receiving the care, and what he or she expects to happen from the care. Therefore, when a treatment is compared to a placebo in clinical trials, the patients should differ only in whether they receive treatment, and not in other aspects.

Not all clinical trials compare an active treatment to a placebo. No patient is denied treatment in a clinical trial if there is a standard therapy available that could improve the comfort and survival of the patient.[6]

Here is a simpler example of the placebo effect: have you ever gone to the doctor to get a letter saying you can't go to work because you have a bad cold—and suddenly begun to feel better while sitting in the clinic, leafing through magazines? It's embarrassing, but easy to explain: your mind generates messages to begin the analgesic or healing processes when you accept that you have in fact started on a path to recovery.[7]

Note:

Not all-clinical trial research is the same. Review the article, paper, and text with a healthy skepticism. Look at who is publishing the item in question as research results can be skewed to fit the hypothesis being tested.

For instance, some years ago Vitamin E was being tested and the researchers determined that there was no benefit to be gained by taking it. What the 10-second sound bite from T.V. did not record was that the researchers were using the synthetic DL form of Vitamin E and not the D – natural source. The D natural source is more bio-available (absorbable) form.

In this instance the public were lead to believe that taking Vitamin E was bad because it could cause health challenges.

When thinking of publishing your research the wisest course of action is to go to peer reviewed and evidence based journals.

The following quote is from Molecules of Emotion.

… we scientists measure our success in terms of papers – how many we've published and where they've appeared, in journals considered top of the line, middle of the list, or bottom of the barrel.

…the only real glory comes from seeing your name in print under the title of a paper. Even more thrilling, at times, is seeing your work cited in another scientist's paper, which is significant because it affects your status in the professional hierarchy. Your position is determined by a huge database called the "citation index," a listing of every paper according to the number of times it has been cited.[8]

With more people turning to CAM for disease prevention, treatment, and health promotion, there is a mounting need for scientific research to investigate the safety profiles of popular treatment modalities, establish clinical efficacy for selected indications, and develop proper educational and training modules for clinicians with patients using CAM. An important area that is lacking focus is an inclusive guide for physicians, CAM practitioners, and patients regarding advice and communication pertaining to CAM use.[9]

There is a wonderful little book "Healing, Intention and Energy Medicine" edited by Wayne B. Jonas and Cindy C. Crawford. The authors have designed a research project to look at all the credible scientific research, which has been done on Energy medicine, spiritual healing and prayer.

In the Appendix 2, Crawford and Jones have provided the reader with a stellar bibliography. It is broken down into categories: randomized clinical studies, basic and laboratory research, reviews, systematic reviews, and meta-analyses, observational studies and non-randomized clinical trials and others (includes: opinions, claims, anecdotes, letters to editors, commentaries, critiques, and meeting reports). This section is almost 50 pages and get out your magnifying glass as the font may be 8 point.

It is hoped that the authors could produce an updated version of this book, as the initial publishing date was 2003, and there has been a lot of research done on this topic of late.

Case Reports

Patient/client case reports are starting to carry some weight in peer reviewed medical journals. With this in mind here is a brief outline as to what the report should contain.

Summary of stages in preparation of background information for a case report:

Identify a suitable patient

Search the literature for similar cases

Obtain consent from the patient or their appointed guardian

Collect information from the patient's case history, examinations and test results

Summary of items to include in a case report

Introduction

Case report history

examination

examination findings

investigations

results of investigations

treatment intervention used

outcome of treatment

Discussion

why you selected this patient for your case report

what the literature reports about similar cases

how rare is this condition?

what is the scientific explanation for this condition?

what is the cause of this condition?

why did you choose you intervention?

how did your intervention influence the outcome for the patient?

what are the standard interventions for this condition?

what are your recommendations for future treatment for this condition?

what lessons can be learned from this case report?

Conclusion

References

Acknowledgements

Additional information[10]

For a more detailed understanding of case reports see the appendix document titled "How to write a case report" by Laine H. McCarthy, MLIS; Kathryn E.H. Reilly, MD, MPH

http://www.stfm.org/fmhub/Fullpdf/march00/fd2.pdf (as of August 2009)

Soap notes

Subjective: The client's subjective complaints and symptoms that are in the client's own words or may have been discussed by the prescribing physician. This includes all the things the client tells you about how they are feeling, past history, present symptoms, limitations in their lives due to the injury, what makes them feel better or worse, and details about the initial onset of the problem or injury. It is often helpful to ask the client to rate their pain or discomfort on a level 1-10 with 10 being the worst. If you do this each time, you will be able to see improvements or setbacks.

Ask specific questions as to the location, intensity, duration and frequency of the pain or discomfort. Have the client point to the specific area on their body or body chart. Ask how painful is it? How long have they had it? Hours? Weeks? Months? Longer? Has it been worse or better? What makes it worse or better? How often do they get it? Every day? Once a week?

Asking specific questions will lead to a clearer picture of the problem/injury you are treating.

Objective: This is the observations of the practitioner and what techniques were done during the session. This includes visual observations and what you feel in the body of the client. Include things you observe about the clients posture, patterns, movement, weakness, level of tension in the tissues, spasms in muscles, joint movement, color/temperature of skin and breathing patterns.

You can also test the range of motion in different areas and keep track of their improvement or changing patterns.

Some common findings are defined below:

Hypertonicity: involuntarily tight or contracted muscle; excess muscle tone; the tension of the resting muscle is unusually high.

Spasm: involuntary contraction of a muscle as a protective response to an injury or trauma.

Trigger point: specific point that refers pain
Adhesion/scar tissue: the resulting tissue from the wound healing process causing a restriction in resiliency of the tissue

Assessment: As most bodyworkers or massage therapists are not allowed to diagnose conditions, this is to report the immediate results of the session. At the end of the session reanalyze the posture and range of motion. Make notes on any changes in symptoms. Indicate how much change happened- mild, moderate or significant change. Use as many descriptive words as possible.

Most insurance companies will take this information into consideration when paying for the treatment. This is what is telling them if the client is getting better and is the treatment worth it.

Plan: Suggest a treatment frequency and things that need to be addressed in the future. Include any self care instructions you gave to the client, special requests by the client, or reminders for the next session.[11]

This topic is discussed more in Chapter 6.

Chapter Review:

The value of quality research on CAM therapies is greatly needed. Depending on the kind of research done would dictate the methodology and reporting of results: double blind placebo controlled or a case study report.

The more that CAM specialists can show the efficacy, low cost and lack of harm these therapies provide, the more these therapies can be integrated into standard western allopathic medical practice.

Chapter 4

Ethics

*Advice is like snow – the softer it falls, the longer it dwells upon and
the deeper it sinks into the mind.*
Samuel Taylor Coleridge[1]

Our patients and clients have driven the movement towards
patient centred care. They talk to friends or other family
members about their health, discussing what is working or alter-
natively what is not. Then there is the influence of television talk
shows like Oprah, Ellen Degeneres and let's not forget about the
Internet.

Most patients use CAM with, rather than instead of, conventional medicine. Most patients use CAM regularly, rather than
as an isolated encounter, and do so for those chronic conditions conventional medicine has been less than successful at
treating, such as musculoskeletal pain or dysfunction,
headaches, chronic or recurring pain, anxiety and depression,
or for potentially terminal conditions such as cancer or HIV.
CAM is used by all age groups, and is typically used by the
more educated, those willing to pay out of pocket, and those
willing to tell their physicians when asked.[2]

Americans spent $33.9 billion out-of-pocket on comple-
mentary and alternative medicine (CAM) over the previous
12 months, according to a 2007 government survey.[1] CAM is a
group of diverse medical and health care systems, practices,
and products such as herbal supplements, meditation, chiropractic, and acupuncture that are not generally considered to
be part of conventional medicine. CAM accounts for approxi-

mately 1.5 percent of total health care expenditures ($2.2 trillion[2]) and 11.2 percent of total out-of-pocket expenditures (conventional out-of-pocket: $286.6 billion[2] and CAM out-of-pocket: $33.9 billion[1]) on health care in the United States.

Approximately 38 percent of adults use some form of CAM for health and wellness or to treat a variety of diseases and conditions, according to data from the 2007 National Health Interview Survey (NHIS).[3] The CAM component of the NHIS was developed by the National Institutes of Health's (NIH) National Center for Complementary and Alternative Medicine (NCCAM) and the National Center for Health Statistics (NCHS) part of the Centers for Disease Control and Prevention. The data provide estimates of the cost of CAM use, the frequency of visits made to CAM practitioners, and frequency of purchases of self-care CAM therapies.

It is our clients's search for knowledge, wanting to know and understand the nature of their latest illness that drives them to question everything. We know that Doctors may not always have time to research what is the most recent development on say the cancer front, or Alzheimer's. So we, the general public, in our efforts to assist the process and wanting to discuss with our health care providers a CAM treatment to see if it is genuine or not, even take our research - the reports into the doctor's office.

In 1997 D.M. Eisenberg wrote an article in the Annals of Internal Medicine listing the five main reasons why patients use CAM:

1. For health promotion and disease prevention.
2. Conventional therapies have been exhausted.
3. Conventional therapies are of indeterminate effectiveness or are commonly associated with side effects or significant risks.
4. No conventional therapy is known to relieve the patient's

condition.

5. The conventional approach is perceived to be emotionally or spiritually without benefit.[3]

Initially the medical community were like the parents of 1950s teens at the beginning of rock and roll. Maybe if we don't pay any attention, it will die out this is just the latest fad.

Well, just like rock and roll music, the alternative health sector has not gone away: it is slowly evolving into Complementary or Integrative health.

This change of name is more than just having to choose between two different styles of health promotion. There is starting to be a change in attitudes too. There have been numerous surveys done regarding the use of Complementary and Alternative (CAM) therapies. It is a growing field due to the empowerment our patients and clients feel, they are taking responsibility for their health.

There was a time not too long ago during the 1990s when more forward thinking Allopathically trained doctors wanted to talk to or learn more about complementary therapies. Those doctors were cautioned and criticized not only by local medical examining boards but also by colleagues for wanting to know about these other forms of therapy.

In addition to these forward thinking conventional doctors, it has been the Chiropractors, Naturopaths, Homeopaths, Acupuncturists and Traditional Chinese Medicine practitioners who have been called quacks and purveyors of snake oil. And any research done in CAM therapies is a waste of taxpayers' dollars.

The web site "Quackwatch" does not have anything good to say about CAM therapies, in fact the site tells the public to stay away.

While the next paragraph does not necessarily deal with Allopathic medicine and CAM, it is encouraging to see that some alliances are happening within some health professions in the allopathic field. There are no CAM therapies included in this list. The website does outline the qualifications a health college or organization would have to fulfill in order to be accepted.

The Ontario government the Ministry of Health and Long-term care formed in 1991 the Health Professions Regulatory Advisory Council (HPRAC) to promote *"Mechanisms to Facilitate and Support Interprofessional Collaboration among Health Colleges and Regulated Health Professionals.*

HPRAC provides independent policy advice to the Minister of Health and Long-term Care on matters related to the regulation of health professions in Ontario.[4]

The Health Professions Regulatory Advisory Council (HPRAC) was established with the introduction of the Regulated Health Professions Act, 1991 (RHPA).

Under the legislation, HPRAC has a statutory mandate to advise the Minister on:

Whether to regulate or de-regulate health professions;

Suggested amendments to the *RHPA* and related Acts and their regulations;

Matters concerning the quality assurance programs of health professional colleges;

Any matter related to the regulation of health professionals referred by the Minister.

The Council also has a statutory duty to monitor Colleges' Patient Relations Programs.

The Council is comprised of seven public members who are appointed by the Lieutenant-Governor in Council to provide policy recommendations to the Minister. The Council endeavours to be independent of stakeholders, and to provide well-documented proposals in the formulation of public policy for the Minister's consideration.[5]

Research in to the safety and effectiveness of Complementary therapies will assist everyone in understanding how CAM therapies work. The more data that comes in, the less frightening this modality will become, and in turn an easier integration with mainstream medicine.

CAM has certainly become a permanent part of the health care culture and landscape as the borders between conventional medicine and CAM begin to blur. The results are numerous clinical, economic, ethical, legal, and social issues associated with not only the increased interest in the use of CAM, but a re-evaluation of conventional medicine as well.[6]

In the United States a number of medical schools have recognized that Complementary health is here to stay. The front line Doctors (General Practitioners) are starting to identify that the communication between themselves and their patients is starting to suffer, because they were unaware about complementary health. So that has led to courses and the development of course curricula at medical institutions like Harvard to address this issue.

See Appendix 3 —"Suggested Curriculum Guidelines on Complementary and Alternative Medicine: Recommendations of the Society of Teachers of Family Medicine Group on Alternative Medicine".

Authors: Benjamin Kligler, MD, MPH; Andrea Gordon, MD; Marian Stuart, PhD; Victor Sierpina, MD

The suggested guidelines, core competencies, and recommendations that the Allopathic community is looking at are: 1) Attitudes and Understanding, 2) Knowledge, 3) Research and Critical Evaluation, and 4) Communication Skills.[7]

With this merging of allopathic and complementary

medicines we are creating a new paradigm called Integrative Medicine.

As exciting as this new field is, there can some growing pains expected. Some allopathic doctors may steadfastly believe that CAM is a waste of money to research. Others sceptics may believe this CAM stuff is nothing more than the placebo effect. At the other end of the spectrum practitioners in the CAM field may be threatened by a perceived notion that they are being squeezed out of the marketplace.

A British report about integration, based on the views of directors of public health and representatives of general practitioner National Health Service fund-holding consortiums, found the following five criteria were most frequently thought to be necessary for integration:

1. Effectiveness
2. Positive outcome studies
3. Cost effectiveness
4. Recognized accreditation procedures and professional standards
5. Availability of qualified practitioners[8]

It is for that very reason that CAM practitioners need to become professional in our chosen scopes of practice. We need to speak with one common voice and no longer be fractured by our diverse viewpoints in our chosen field.

In the book Professionalism and Ethics in Complementary and Alternative Medicine, the authors John Crellin and Fernando Ania discuss this very issue.

"Polarized views and factionalism are common as reflected in the plethora of complementary/alternative medicine organizations and educational standards. Although discord can be a sign of growth—in fact, some see it as a step toward professionalization—it raises concerns inside and outside the movement. Those striving for professionalism, at least licensing and uniform standards of practice, often find themselves at loggerheads with those who want no regulation.[9]

If your practice is low key and work is just done on yourself and your family (private) some of the following information may not apply to you, but may be of casual interest. However, if you do have clients coming to your home for Reiki sessions then the information on the subsequent pages are important for you too.

In a private practice the concern about filling out paper work — client consent forms are really not important, unless you want to keep track of how the sessions are progressing.

Things are much more flexible when you are practicing privately at home. The massage table may be your kitchen table with the mattress pad you use for camping, the living room couch, a family member's bed. Or if the time being spent on doing Reiki is small, it may be those few precious and quiet moments between rushing off to do this or that.

Taking the time to use Reiki at these moments can assist in calming down the intensity of a frantic busy day.

A public home practice is just a little more formal. Then again it all depends on how much effort you are willing to spend building a practice.

In the beginning practicing on family and friends is an excellent way for you to practice this new skill and a nice way to spread the word as to what Reiki is about. Once you have exhausted this avenue, it may be time to expand your sphere of influence.

Aside from hanging a shingle on your house saying REIKI PRACTICED HERE, business cards or a flyer might be a better option. Note: hanging out a shingle may be in contravention of your local by-laws, please check with your municipal government **first**.

If you're just looking to do a few cards then going to your

local office supply store like Staples, Grand & Toy and etc., to pick up a blank package of card sheets will work just fine.

Needing to have more of a professional look but are not ready yet to go to a printer, then contact Vista print on the Internet. You can pick a style that suits your needs at an affordable price.

When possible get a professional head shot taken of you. This picture could be used on your business card, on a brochure or post it to your web site. Remember some clients want to see and "get an energetic feel" for what you would be like to work with.

As you ease yourself into the exciting profession of Reiki practitioner you discover that clients are expecting a more polished and professional you to greet them at the door.

The medical community is regulated by their own professional colleges, which are accountable to the provincial or state government. I.e.: the College of Physicians and Surgeons, Ontario College of Nursing, College of Chiropodists (and Podiatrists), etc.

For others the provincial or state government sets guidelines for an approved program standard. These two examples can be classified as statutory regulation.

In the Complementary health field we do not have a body regulating what is taught, the number of class hours or how a practitioner should behave towards a client.

At the moment it is up to the discretion of the Reiki practitioner if they wish to join the Canadian Reiki Association. (CRA) Most Reiki practitioners have not joined, for some it is the issue of cost, others may not feel they are getting value for becoming a member. As a self-regulating body the CRA will need time to lay a strong foundation on which to build a credible organization.

Crellin and Anin in their research discovered that the public would like Complementary practitioners held to the same high standards that physicians are required to maintain. These would be "possessing the traditional virtues of the 'good' physician (e.g., honesty, truthfulness, compassion, etc.), but also that physicians fulfill such roles as communicator, scientist, healer, health advocate, team player, and gatekeeper."[10]

In addition to the items mentioned in the British report on page 56 the public is also concerned about curricula content and continuing education. Once again the discussion revolves around standards. While most Reiki folks are not from a medical background like nursing, the public feels that we would better understand their health issues if we knew about anatomy, physiology and biochemistry. As to how much we should know of these topics Crellin and Anin are not clear but they do suggest we have solid basic science knowledge:

1. aid a complementary/alternative practitioner's ability to understand the conventional medical treatment a patient may be having;
2. increase an 'index of suspicion' of multisystem disease and of cases that should be referred to others;
3. help to recognize possible incompatibilities between two treatments; and
4. ensure that practitioners constantly evaluate research and the changing relationships between complementary/alternative care and medical science.[11]

Arti Prasad, MD and Mariebeth B. Velásquez, BS have looked at this issue too they feel that CAM practitioners have limited knowledge in the following areas:

1. Concepts of conventional medicine and ways to integrate them with CAM
2. Natural health care products: safety, efficacy, interactions with herbs, drugs, and food
3. Latest research in CAM
4. Access to reliable databases, websites, books, journals, continuing education, and other resources on CAM.[12]

If a physician refers a client to you and they start asking the following questions, don't get hostile and feel like you're being put under a microscope, the client is just doing what they have been asked.

Table 4 – What to Ask a CAM Practitioner[13]

1. Is this particular therapy a recognized treatment for my disorder?
2. What is your educational and training background?
3. Can you share some research on the safety and efficacy of this treatment?
4. Do you have experience and success treating my symptoms or disorder?
5. How many patients have you successfully treated using this particular therapy?
6. What is the length and cost of the proposed treatment?
7. What are your other professional competencies?
8. What other kinds of problems do you treat?
9. How many patients do you see in a day?
10. How comfortable do you feel working in collaboration with my primary care physician?
11. How would you communicate with my physician?
12. How do you assess the effectiveness of this treatment?
13. What is the stopping point in the treatment protocol?
14. Are patient education or professional references available?

You would have to agree these are pretty heavy-duty questions. Take some time and become comfortable answering them. If necessary role-play with a friend, when given objections, know how will you handle them.

This manual is a beginning point for those of us in Reiki to become familiar with the terminology of the medical community. The rest of this chapter is devoted to ethics, and then next chapter is basic anatomy and physiology.

What exactly does having a code of conduct mean?

The dictionary gives a number of definitions but all seem to apply equally.

Noun

1. behaviour; a way of acting
2. the action or manner of directing or managing (business, war, etc.)
3. (archaic) leading, guidance

This definition could be applied to all the interactions we experience with one another: our children's schools, sports teams, business dealings and healthcare professionals. In essence we agree to work in fairness and honestly together, sharing the work evenly. I realize this is not the case in all things, but this is our working definition.

When we work with a client no matter the setting whether at home, in our clinic, at hospice, in a hospital or wherever, these are the ground rules by which we work.

The following are the guidelines most Integrative Practitioners would follow. However, based on the professional associations you may join. the exact wording of Code of Ethics and Conduct may vary.

There are other organizations you can join, make sure you take time to read the membership criteria not all groups have the same guidelines.

Here is a guideline I developed after reviewing samples in the CAM field.

Integrative Healing

Statement of Ethics and Conduct

1. The Integrative Practitioner will conduct their practice in accordance with the principles outlined per their modality.
2. All fees will be disclosed to the client prior to their session.
3. The client has the right to accept or refuse any form of treatment. I the practitioner also have the right to accept or refuse a client for reasons of my personal safety and/or other reasons, providing those reasons are not based upon sex, race, religion, disability, sexual orientation, political belief or personal wealth.
4. I will advise clients that this modality is a complementary therapy and recommend that clients seek treatment and/or continue with treatment by qualified practitioners for any medical condition. I will make appropriate referral of a client to suitably qualified health practitioners if required.
5. When the client is a child under the age of majority, a parent or legal guardian will be present during the session.
6. In accordance with PIPEDA I will keep all client information in a safe, secure, private location. I will not share any information without written consent from the client. When client information is no longer needed, it will be shredded and destroyed.
7. I will ensure that all interpersonal transactions between the client and me are non-exploitive and essential to her/his care.
8. I acknowledge that this therapeutic relationship may increase the rapport between the client and myself

therefore I will keep all information in strict confidence.

9. I will focus on the needs of the client and will refrain from discussing my personal issues with the client.

10. I will not use my modality as a basis for psychotherapy, spiritual or other counseling, unless I have the training and qualifications to do so, as well as permission of the client.

11. I will dress in a professional manner conducive to the holistic service being provided and be neat and clean in my own personal hygiene.

12. The use of alcohol and/or mind altering substances is strictly forbidden when practicing or teaching any Integrative Healing modality.

13. I will maintain the highest integrity, keeping the interest of the client foremost, and I will conduct all sessions in a manner that upholds the professional nature of my modality.

14. I will strive for self-improvement and seek to enhance my abilities by means of further education and training.

15. I will regularly evaluate my strengths, limitations and levels of effectiveness.

16. I understand that, should Integrative Healing receive any complaints about my sessions, or my conduct, I will be notified of that complaint. If, after due process of investigation, a mutually acceptable resolution of any associated problems cannot be achieved, Integrative Healing has the right to withdraw my name from the list of members.

It is understood that Integrative Healing is hereby saved harmless from liability of any kind whatsoever for the actions or lack thereof of its Integrative Practitioners in fulfillment of their association membership.

I understand my signature is considered legal and binding and that it verifies I have completed this form completely and honestly.

Signed _____ Dated _____

The Hospice Association of Ontario (HAO) held their annual conference (2011) and Marianne Tavares and Cindy Webber presented a workshop on Complementary Therapy Standards. These ladies are on a committee to look at the requirements CAM practitioners should have when offering their services in Hospice Palliative care settings.

The following draft – Standard 7 out of 12 – was given to attendees at the workshop. Marianne has given verbal permission to reprint.

HAO Complementary Therapy Standards[14]
Standard 7 (draft)

7. **The hospice has written information for therapists and practitioners on the ethical behaviour and practice expected**.
Indicators
The written information indicates that the therapist/practitioner meets the standard by acting at all times to such a manner as to:
a. Safeguard and promote the interests and well-being of clients.
b. Justify the trust and confidence of clients.
c. Uphold and enhance the good standing and reputation of their complementary therapy profession.
d. Uphold and enhance the good standing of the hospice.
e. Ensure there are no conflict of interest issues related to the delivery of the therapy.

Therapists and practitioners are made aware that they are

personally accountable for their practice and in the exercise of that professional accountability must:

f.   Be willing to sign a statement that they agree to abide by the hospice ethical standards and all relevant policies and protocols.

g.   Ensure that no action or omission on their part is detrimental to the interests, condition or safety of clients.

h.   Maintain and improve their professional knowledge and competence.

i.   Recognize the limits of their professional competence.

j.   Make no claims for their treatment other than to enhance the quality of life of clients.

k.   Communicate and provide information in a way that clients can understand and which is not overwhelming in the client's condition.

l.   Work in partnership with clients, foster their independence and respect the treatment choices they make.

m.   Provide complementary therapy or modality only with the agreement of and as directed by the client, caregiver or hospice and in accordance with hospice policy.

n.   Respond to clients' need for care, irrespective of gender, age, race, ethnicity, disability, sexuality, socio-economic status, culture or religious beliefs.

o.   Maintain professional boundaries and avoid any abuse of their privileged relationship with clients and of the privileged access allowed to the client's person, property or residence.

p.   Avoid entering into any personal or other professional relationship with the client without prior discussion with the coordinator of the complementary therapy program.

q.   Avoid any behaviour that may be perceived as seeking to enhance the therapist or practitioner's private practice.

r.   Protect all confidential information concerning clients obtained in the course of professional practice and make disclosures only with consent or within the policy of confidentiality as practiced within the hospice, subject to the limits of confidentiality in compliance with current legislation.

s. Refuse any gift, favour or hospitality from clients currently in their care which might be interpreted as seeking to exert influence to obtain preferential consideration.

t. Work in a collaborative and cooperative manner with the interdisciplinary team and others involved in providing care.

u. Recognize and respect the role and contribution of colleagues within conventional medicine and other complementary therapists or practitioners; for example when interacting with a client do not criticize or question any other colleague's approach and/or decisions.

v. Report to an appropriate person or authority any circumstances which could jeopardize or compromise safety or standards of practice, including the fitness of themselves or a colleague to practice, while having regard to the physical, psychological and social effects on clients.

April 2011

Cultural Competency

Another aspect of being ethical is being cognizant and having Cultural Competency.

Personal communication with Dr. Joan Lesmond, RN, BScN, MSN, Ed.D at St. Elizabeth Health Care Foundation, Markham, ON December 2009

Why is cultural competence important?

It is an opportunity to meet people where they are at with regards to their health and their culture.

It increases awareness with regards to the person who is being treated. By taking the time to get to know the client - the client/patient a relationship is formed which can truly meet their needs.

Cultural competence looks beyond "culture as ethnicity" to explore the complexities of individual cultural identities: For example: the tip of an iceberg – what is really underneath?

Culturally congruent care delivery – policy and procedures, training, skills, etc. All these elements help to create an experience of warm care. This warm care is one of the people tasks that connects us and creates relationships.

Explain how the current health model could impact a patient/clients' health?

The current model is striving to make the patient/client experience the best ever through looking at policies, procedures, skills, knowledge.

Client's/Patients values and belief system influence their perceptions of health and learned patterns of response to illness and treatment.

Dr. Lesmond suggests that when we take the history of the client it includes:

What bothers you about Integrative Health,(CAM Therapies) do you have any concerns, how does your culture interact with this?

This is a presentation Dr. Lesmond gave at the North Simcoe Muskoka Palliative Care Conference in Midland, ON., dealing with defining and developing cultural competency.

The following definitions are from the presentation handouts:

Culture:

is learned, shared and transmitted values, beliefs, norms and live practices of a particular group that guides thinking decisions and actions in patterned ways. Madeline Leininger (1978)

Culture can best be described as learned from birth; shared dynamic and adapted to certain conditions. Tyler (1874)

Cultural Diversity:

Differences based on gender, class, ability, disability, sexual orientation, race, religion, lifestyle, socioeconomic status, geography, age, education, language, etc.

Ethnoracial differences

Different from the norm versus different from each other

Core value that influences organizational culture

Should do no harm

Cultural Competence

Is a dynamic process of framing assumptions, knowledge and meanings from an individual's background and experience, which is different than our own.

How many of us really take time to understand the background of this person?

Looks beyond "culture as ethnicity to explore the complexities of individual cultural identities".

Builds on cultural sensitivity. The way they would like to be treated.

Is a developmental process that evolves over an extended period.

Cultural Sensitivity vs. Cultural Competence

Awareness, respect for and openness to cultural differences

Understanding of legacies and layers

Translating the awareness into action

Requires skill development

Willingness and ability to take action
Srivasta 2007

Dimensions of Culture Care:

Culture Sensitivity

Culture Knowledge

Culture Resources (finances to support Cultural Competence)

Culturally Congruent Care Delivery

Understanding of Professional Organizational Culture

Understanding of own biases, beliefs, prejudices, values and
culture.

Understanding of issues of power, trust and equity.

Srivastava 2007

Understanding Cultural Implications in Health Care:

Must understand the link between culture – health – illness.

Leininger states that people are born, live, become ill and die
within a cultural belief.

Various cultures have differing beliefs pertaining to health
and illness

Interventions are based on perceived causes, common beliefs
of Heath Care Team reflect their culture of origin, culture of their
profession, and the culture of the North American health and
illness.

Culture encompasses all facets of our lives.

Recognizing Barriers to Effective Care:

Cultural Categorization: overgeneralization, pigeon hole
approach, e.g. African-Canadian, Chinese-Canadian. Each client
is dealt with on a case-by-case basis.

Stereotyping: Ascribing values, attitudes, attributes of a small
number of people to all members in the group

Ethnocentrism: Paternalistic = My approach is more desirable

Cultural Imposition: Imposing values, beliefs, behaviour

upon another culture, e.g. traditional health care system.

Privacy Legislation

Compliance guidelines for your business

The federal (Canadian) Personal Information Protection and Electronic Documents Act, came into effect on January 1, 2004. As a result, all businesses are subject to new stringent guidelines regarding the collection, storage and disclosure of private and personal information collected on individuals. Failure to comply with the Act can result in lawsuits and the awarding of punitive damages.

Businesses located in Quebec are already regulated under provincial privacy legislation (for information on Quebec's legislation go to the website for La Commission d'accès à l'information du Québec **http://www.cai.gouv.qc.ca/**).

The following is a brief outline of how the privacy legislation affects your business:[15]

WHAT IS PERSONAL INFORMATION?

The Privacy legislation defines personal information as: age, name, weight, height, medical records, ID numbers, income, ethnic origin, blood type, opinions, evaluations, comments, social status, employee files, disciplinary action, credit records, loan records, existence of a dispute between a consumer and a merchant and intentions (for example, to acquire goods or services, or change jobs.)

WHAT THE ACT COVERS

Accountability: The Act states that organizations must have a documented Privacy policy, and appoint an internal Privacy Expert/Commissioner who is knowledgeable about the legislation and able to train persons who will be collecting, using, or disclosing personal information.

Identification of Purposes: Individuals must be informed of the purpose for the collection, and how the information might be used or disclosed to other outside organizations.

Consent: There are three types of consent that can be used, A. Express Consent/Permission (Opt-in), B. Negative Option (Opt-out), and C. Implied Consent. Information of a more sensitive nature (health, medical, financial) will require stronger methods of obtaining consent (Please refer to the Privacy Commissioner web site for a detailed description of these options.)

Limiting Collection: Gather only the information that is necessary for the identified purposes.

Limit Use, Disclosure, and Retention: Personal information must only be used for the purposes for which consent has been given. Only keep the information for as long as it is necessary.

Accuracy: Personal Information should be accurate. Processes/procedures must be put in place for persons to flag and rectify inaccuracies in their own personal information.

Safeguards: Measures must be taken to ensure that personal information is secured, such as locked cabinets, electronic firewalls, and limited staff access.

Openness: Privacy policies and practices should be available in a public document or web site.

Individual Access: Ability to inform individuals how their information was collected, used and disclosed, including a list of with whom their information has been shared.

Provide Recourse: Privacy policies should describe complaint resolution procedures.

COMPLIANCE TIPS:

Obtain consent when collecting personal information from a customer. Consent can be obtained in person, by phone, by mail, by fax or via the Internet.

Make sure clients fully understand how their information will be used.

Define your purposes for collecting data as clearly and narrowly as possibly. This allows less data to be collected.

Limit who has access to personal information.

Protect personal information against loss or theft. Store it in a locked cabinet, using a program that only a few employees have access to, use an encryption program for electronic data, use passwords on files.

Let the customer know why you need to collect the data.

Inform customers, clients and employees that you have policies and practices for the management of personal information. Make these policies available and easy to understand.

Develop customer complaint procedures and investigate all complaints received.

WHAT THE ACT DOESN'T COVER

- The Collection, use or disclosure of personal information by federal government organizations listed in the Privacy Act;
- Provincial or territorial governments and their agents;
- An employee's name, title, business address or telephone number;
- An individual's collection, use or disclosure of personal information strictly for personal purposes (e.g. personal greeting card list); and,
- The collection, use or disclosure of personal information solely for journalistic, artistic or literary purposes.

WHERE TO GET MORE INFORMATION

For up to date announcements and useful links to privacy related sites please reference the CFIB Privacy page on the National Affairs website: **http://www.cfib.ca/legis/national/ Privacy.asp**

To access the official documents or to receive more detailed information on the issue please refer to Resource Centre on the Privacy Commissioner of Canada's website **http://www.priv com.gc.ca or call 1-800-282-1376.**

PROVINCIAL LEGISLATION

The federal privacy legislation meets international requirements allowing Canadian firms to do business internationally. Although the federal Act covers all organizations across Canada, some provinces have decided to draft legislation which exceeds the scope of the federal legislation. Currently only Quebec has passed private sector privacy legislation, however legislation is in the works for Ontario, British Columbia and Alberta.

Quebec
La Commission d'accès à l'information du Québec **http://www.cai.gouv.qc.ca/** or call toll free **1-888-528-7741.**

In the United States the Department of Health and Human Services, has its own policy.

Medical Privacy-National Standards to Protect the Privacy of Personal Health Information.

The Privacy Rule

The HIPAA Privacy Rule establishes national standards to protect individuals' medical records and other personal health information and applies to health plans, health care clearinghouses, and those health care providers that conduct certain health care transactions electronically. The Rule requires appropriate safeguards to protect the privacy of personal health information, and sets limits and conditions on the uses and disclosures that may be made of such information without patient authorization. The Rule also gives patients rights over their health information, including rights to examine and obtain a copy of their health records, and to request corrections.

http://www.hhs.gov/ocr/privacy/hipaa/administrative/privacy rule/index.html

In the United Kingdom you need to get in touch with the Information Commissioner's Office (ICO). There are a couple of sites that will be of interest to you:

http://www.ico.gov.uk/for_organisations/topic_specific_guide s/health.aspx

http://www.ico.gov.uk/for_organisations/data_protection_gui de.aspx

For other countries who may be reading this manual I strongly urge you to check local legislation, in order to safe guard yourself from being on the wrong side of the law.

This may be a good time to discuss the distinction between having a public and private practice.

Having a public practice requires the practitioner to do their work a little differently, such as being aware of governmental regulations regarding handling our clients' personal information.

Gone are the days when a practitioner would put all the names gathered from a trade show give-away onto their mailing lists. Now, because of legislation our free draw slips have to ask the potential client if they would like to be included on our mailing lists. It is not a given anymore, the client has the right to say no. If you do email notices the same applies, there must be a link or a way for the client to be removed [opt-out] from your list.

Another item we need to be aware of is client information storage. Aside from holding files in a secure file cabinet, how long do we hold them for?

With Canadian federal income tax by law we are required to hold that taxation year say 2008 for seven years until 2015. Then we can shred it and create some room in our file box for the current years tax return.

How long do allopathic doctors have to keep patient records?

Massage therapists (RMT) have been advised to keep files for 10 years on clients who are legal adults. In the case of minors, massage therapists are required to keep those same files for 10 years after the minor turns 18. So if the minor were three, those files would be kept in safe keeping for 31 years. For some RMT's that could be longer than their years in active practice.

Just something else we need to think about. I would say anywhere between 7 and 10 years.

Scenario 1

New client has called you and wishes to have a reiki session in your office.

When they arrive once the exchange of greetings has been done, ask them to complete the Consent release form.

On the form it asks if they have any questions about Reiki, if so now is the time to answer them.

Enquire if there is anything that they would specifically like to work on. (i.e.: sore shoulder, digestive upset, etc.)

Proceed with reiki session.

Scenario 2

New client has arrived a mother and child for a reiki session.

When they arrive once the exchange of greetings has been done, ask the mother to complete the Consent release form, if the child is under the age of 18.

If you have talked to the mother beforehand ask her to bring some of the child's favourite relaxing music, as this can help reduce the child's nervousness.

Try to explain Reiki to the child in a way that they would understand, as sometimes they can be quite nervous as to what it is you are going to do.

In all instances it is quite ok and expected, for the parent or guardian to remain in the room.

Depending on the age of the child they may not be able to sit or lie still for extended periods of time. Frequent sessions may be more effective than one long one. You may want to adjust your fees accordingly.

Scenario 3

New client telephones and asks if you make house calls as they have someone who is bed-ridden and cannot come to your clinic.

First you need to decide if you're going to accept the person as a client and then discuss your fee. Is it going to be an hourly rate and then mileage on top, or are you going to charge a flat fee, which will include both?

Do you need a copy or need to see the Power of Attorney form for personal care?

When you arrive and once the exchange of greetings has been done, ask if the person you are speaking with is the legal guardian to complete the Consent release form. Should this person not be the guardian, you will need their consent before you can begin working on this new client.

In all cases remember that confidentiality is of great importance to your client. Transport this documentation in portfolio or binder, which is lockable. If these files are to be stored at your clinic space, invest in a quality filing cabinet that can be locked.

Confidentiality also includes not discussing client information with others unless you have the expressed written permission of your client.

Informed Consent

All health care professionals (doctors, nurses, dentists, chiropractors, massage therapists and you) must discuss the issue of consent with their clients.

Informed consent can be either written or verbal, most times written is sufficient. Although under certain conditions, eg. touching a client's breast area during a session to treat breast cancer, verbal permission is also advisable. In this case, should the client have breast tenderness from surgery not even verbal permission is appropriate. It would be advisable for the practitioner to use the hands-off technique.

Ask your clients to complete a Consent and Release form. In the case of a child or if your client is unable to sign the Consent form have the legal guardian sign the document on their behalf.

In Ontario we have the **Health Care Consent Act, (HCCA)** 1996. Below are some of the highlights, I would encourage you to look at the HCCA, and the web address is listed in the endnotes.

For other provinces and readers living outside of Canada your Ministry or National Department of Health should be able to assist you. Failing that contact your provincial or state Nursing College, this is how I found out about HCCA.

The HCCA defines health practitioner as meaning:

(a)   a member of the College of Audiologists and Speech-Language Pathologists of Ontario,

(b)   a member of the College of Chiropodists of Ontario, including a member who is a podiatrist,

(c)   a member of the College of Chiropractors of Ontario,

(d)   a member of the College of Dental Hygienists of Ontario,

(e)   a member of the Royal College of Dental Surgeons of Ontario,

(f)   a member of the College of Denturists of Ontario,

(g)   a member of the College of Dietitians of Ontario,

(g.0.1) a member of the College of Homeopaths of Ontario,

(g.1)   a member of the College of Kinesiologists of Ontario,

(h)   a member of the College of Massage Therapists of Ontario,

(i)   a member of the College of Medical Laboratory Technologists of Ontario,

(j)   a member of the College of Medical Radiation Technologists of Ontario,

(k)   a member of the College of Midwives of Ontario,

(l)   a member of the College of Nurses of Ontario,

(m)   a member of the College of Occupational Therapists of Ontario,

(n)   a member of the College of Optometrists of Ontario,

(o)   a member of the College of Physicians and Surgeons of Ontario,

(p)   a member of the College of Physiotherapists of Ontario,

(q)   a member of the College of Psychologists of Ontario,

(q.1)   a member of the College of Psychotherapists and Registered Mental Health Therapists of Ontario,

(r)   a member of the College of Respiratory Therapists of Ontario,

(s)   a naturopath registered as a drugless therapist under the *Drugless Practitioners Act*, or

(s)   a member of the College of Naturopaths of Ontario,

The purpose of this legislation is:

(a)   to provide rules with respect to consent to treatment that apply consistently in all settings;

(b)   to facilitate treatment, admission to care facilities, and personal assistance services, for persons lacking the capacity to make decisions about such matters;

(c)   to enhance the autonomy of persons for whom treatment is proposed, persons for whom admission to a care facility is proposed and persons who are to receive personal assistance services by, allowing those who have been found to be incapable to apply to a tribunal for a review of the finding,

(ii)   allowing incapable persons to request that a representative of their choice be appointed by the tribunal for the purpose of making decisions on their behalf concerning treatment, admission to a care facility or personal assistance services, and

(iii)   requiring that wishes with respect to treatment, admission to a care facility or personal assistance services, expressed by persons while capable and after attaining 16 years of age, be adhered to;

(d)   to promote communication and understanding between health practitioners and their patients or clients;

(e)   to ensure a significant role for supportive family members when a person lacks the capacity to make a decision about a treatment, admission to a care facility or a personal assistance service; and

(f)   to permit intervention by the Public Guardian and Trustee only as a last resort in decisions on behalf of incapable persons concerning treatment, admission to a care facility or personal assistance services. 1996, c. 2, Sched. A, s. 1.[16]

Consent to Treatment

No treatment without consent

10. (1) A health practitioner who proposes a treatment for a person shall not administer the treatment, and shall take reasonable steps to ensure that it is not administered, unless,

(a) he or she is of the opinion that the person is capable with respect to the treatment, and the person has given consent; or

(b) he or she is of the opinion that the person is incapable with respect to the treatment, and the person's substitute decision-maker has given consent on the person's behalf in accordance with this Act. 1996, c. 2, Sched. A, s. 10 (1).

Opinion of Board or court governs

(2) If the health practitioner is of the opinion that the person is incapable with respect to the treatment, but the person is found to be capable with respect to the treatment by the Board on an application for review of the health practitioner's finding, or by a court on an appeal of the Board's decision, the health practitioner shall not administer the treatment, and shall take reasonable steps to ensure that it is not administered, unless the person has given consent. 1996, c. 2, Sched. A, s. 10 (2).

Elements of consent

11. (1) The following are the elements required for consent to treatment:

1. The consent must relate to the treatment.
2. The consent must be informed.
3. The consent must be given voluntarily.
4. The consent must not be obtained through misrepresentation or fraud. 1996, c. 2, Sched. A, s. 11 (1).

Informed consent

(2) A consent to treatment is informed if, before giving it,

(a) the person received the information about the matters set out in subsection (3) that a reasonable person in the same circumstances would require in order to make a decision about the treatment; and

(b) the person received responses to his or her requests for additional information about those matters. 1996, c. 2, Sched. A, s. 11 (2).

Same

(3) The matters referred to in subsection (2) are:

1. The nature of the treatment.
2. The expected benefits of the treatment.
3. The material risks of the treatment.
4. The material side effects of the treatment.
5. Alternative courses of action.
6. The likely consequences of not having the treatment. 1996, c. 2, Sched. A, s. 11 (3).

Express or implied

(4) Consent to treatment may be express or implied. 1996, c. 2, Sched. A, s. 11 (4).

Included consent

12. Unless it is not reasonable to do so in the circumstances, a health practitioner is entitled to presume that consent to a treatment includes,

(a) consent to variations or adjustments in the treatment, if the nature, expected benefits, material risks and material side effects of the changed treatment are not significantly different from the nature, expected benefits, material risks and material side effects of the original treatment; and

(b) consent to the continuation of the same treatment in a different setting, if there is no significant change in the expected benefits, material risks or material side effects of the treatment as a result of the change in the setting in which it is administered. 1996, c. 2, Sched. A, s. 12.

Plan of treatment

13. If a plan of treatment is to be proposed for a person, one health practitioner may, on behalf of all the health practitioners involved in the plan of treatment,

(a) propose the plan of treatment;

(b) determine the person's capacity with respect to the treatments referred to in the plan of treatment; and

(c) obtain a consent or refusal of consent in accordance with this Act,

(i) from the person, concerning the treatments with respect to which the person is found to be capable, and

(ii) from the person's substitute decision-maker, concerning the treatments with respect to which the person is found to be incapable. 1996, c. 2, Sched. A, s. 13.

Withdrawal of consent

14. A consent that has been given by or on behalf of the person for whom the treatment was proposed may be withdrawn at any time,

(a) by the person, if the person is capable with respect to the treatment at the time of the withdrawal;

(b) by the person's substitute decision-maker, if the person is incapable with respect to the treatment at the time of the withdrawal. 1996, c. 2, Sched. A, s. 14.

In the event that your client is unable to give their consent to a Reiki session the legislation is quite clear as to how to proceed.

Consent on Incapable Person's Behalf
Consent

List of persons who may give or refuse consent

20. (1) If a person is incapable with respect to a treatment, consent may be given or refused on his or her behalf by a person described in one of the following paragraphs:

1. The incapable person's guardian of the person, if the guardian has authority to give or refuse consent to the treatment.

2. The incapable person's attorney for personal care, if the power of attorney confers authority to give or refuse consent to the treatment.

3. The incapable person's representative appointed by the Board under section 33, if the representative has authority to give or refuse consent to the treatment.

4. The incapable person's spouse or partner.

5. A child or parent of the incapable person, or a children's aid society or other person who is lawfully entitled to give or refuse consent to the treatment in the place of the parent. This paragraph does not include a parent who has only a right of access. If a children's aid society or other person is lawfully entitled to give or refuse consent to the treatment in the place of the parent, this paragraph does not include the parent.

6. A parent of the incapable person who has only a right of access.

7. A brother or sister of the incapable person.

8. Any other relative of the incapable person. 1996, c. 2, Sched. A, s. 20 (1).

Requirements

(2) A person described in subsection (1) may give or refuse consent only if he or she,

(a) is capable with respect to the treatment;

(b) is at least 16 years old, unless he or she is the incapable person's parent;

(c) is not prohibited by court order or separation agreement from having access to the incapable person or giving or refusing consent on his or her behalf;

(d) is available; and

(e) is willing to assume the responsibility of giving or refusing consent. 1996, c. 2, Sched. A, s. 20 (2).

Should a client or their care giver choose to not receive a Reiki session by law they are within their legal rights.

Principles for giving or refusing consent

21. (1) A person who gives or refuses consent to a treatment on an incapable person's behalf shall do so in accordance with the following principles:

1. If the person knows of a wish applicable to the circumstances that the incapable person expressed while capable and after attaining 16 years of age, the person shall give or refuse consent in accordance with the wish.

2. If the person does not know of a wish applicable to the circumstances that the incapable person expressed while capable and after attaining 16 years of age, or if it is impossible to comply with the wish, the person shall act in the incapable person's best interests. 1996, c. 2, Sched. A, s. 21 (1).

Best interests

(2) In deciding what the incapable person's best interests are, the person who gives or refuses consent on his or her behalf shall take into consideration,

(a) the values and beliefs that the person knows the incapable person held when capable and believes he or she would still act on if capable;

(b) any wishes expressed by the incapable person with respect to the treatment that are not required to be followed under paragraph 1 of subsection (1); and

(c) the following factors:

1. Whether the treatment is likely to,

i. improve the incapable person's condition or well-being,

ii. prevent the incapable person's condition or well-being from deteriorating, or

iii. reduce the extent to which, or the rate at which, the incapable person's condition or well-being is likely to deteriorate.

2. Whether the incapable person's condition or well-being is likely to improve, remain the same or deteriorate without the treatment.

3. Whether the benefit the incapable person is expected to obtain from the treatment outweighs the risk of harm to him or her.

4. Whether a less restrictive or less intrusive treatment would be as beneficial as the treatment that is proposed. 1996, c. 2, Sched. A, s. 21 (2).[17]

It is up to you as the practitioner to inform your client of the benefits and the risks of having a reiki session and also of not having a reiki session.

"...it is also a professional/ethical responsibility to serve the best interests of patients by presenting all information and establishing boundaries of competence."[18]

Some of the benefits are listed below (but not limited to):

Relaxation, stress reduction, stimulation of immune function, reduction of anxiety, help manage side effects from pharmaceutical drugs, and can enhance rapport between client and health provider and lastly there is no risk of overdose.

The risks of not having a reiki session would be missing out on the opportunity to experience this healing art. It is also advisable to share with a client to keep an eye on the dosage of their pharmaceutical medication. For instance, if a client is taking something for anxiety and having Reiki assists them in feeling less anxious, the client may want to discuss with their health care provider about lowering the dosage. In the event that an allopathic practitioner referred your client to you, get the clients permission before sharing anything like reporting observations from your files.

With respect to safety, the National Center for Complementary and Alternative Medicine (NCCAM) states that there have been no reported negative effects from Reiki in any of the research studies. While Reiki is a hands-on healing art, it is still possible to experience Reiki with hands not touching the body.

Reiki appears to be generally safe, and no serious side effects have been reported.[19]

In a medical facility in England, [College Surgery, Devon] Tim Harlow did an experiment with having a healer working in the clinic [initially one then added a second] on cases. In a paper titled "The impact of healing in a clinical setting"; this was one of the comments. "A major factor which should be emphasized at this point was the complete lack of adverse effects due to healing. For an effective and relatively inexpensive treatment to seem to be entirely free of adverse side-effects is remarkable."20

If you are considering using your client's condition as a candidate for journal publication as a case report, your client will have to give consent. The previous chapter gave an overview on how to write a case report.

Integrative Healing – Consent and Release Form

Client's Full Name:_____

Date of Birth: _____   Gender: Female _____   Male _____

Client Address: _____

Telephone: Home ( )_____   Work (____)_____ (ext)_____

Reiki Practitioners do not diagnose conditions, nor do they prescribe substances or perform medical treatment, nor interfere with the treatment of a licensed medical professional. It is recommended that I see a licensed physician, or licensed health care professional for any physical or psychological ailment or condition I may have.

All information collected will be kept strictly confidential unless it needs to be shared with the other members of a health care team or required by law. Your written permission will be required to release any information.

Client signature: _____

Date: _____

How did you hear about us: _____

Would you be interested in receiving our healthy newsletter   Yes_____   No _____

Your email address: _____

Personal Details:
Lifestyle: Active _____   Sedentary _____

Do you follow a Wellness programme: Healthy food _____   Exercise _____

Do you take time for yourself? _____

What are you hoping to achieve from your session today? _____

Health History: please indicate conditions you are experiencing or have experienced:

Respiratory	Other conditions	Women
__chronic cough	__loss of sensation	__pregnancy (due:_____)
__shortness of breath	__diabetes	__menstrual discomfort
__bronchitis	__multiple sclerosis	__menopause
__asthma	__epilepsy	
__emphysema	__cancer	
	__arthritis	
Cardiovascular	**Head/neck**	**Soft tissue/joint pain or**

discomfort

__high blood pressure   __vision problems   __neck
__low blood pressure   __vision loss   __upper back
__congestive heart failure   __ear problems   __mid back
__phlebitis   __hearing loss   __low back
__stroke/CVA   __headaches   __shoulders
__pacemaker   __migraines   __arms
__heart disease   __sinus   __legs
__varicose veins   __knees
                                                      __other
                                                      __ pins, wires, artificial limbs

Infections	Sleep	Stress	Digestive
__hepatitis	__restless	__work	
__TB	__insomnia	__other	__gas, bloating
__HIV			

Excretory   **Skin**
__1 movement/day   __herpes   __athlete's foot   __Allergies (respiratory,
                                                                  skin, food inc. nuts)
__ more than one   __warts   __contact dermatitis   __sensitivity to perfume,
                                                                          smells

Any other medical condition not mentioned above:_____
_____

Are you currently under the care of your Family Physician or Specialist? Yes_____   No ___
If yes, please elaborate _____

Are you taking prescription medication?   Yes _____   No _____
If yes, which ones _____

Are you currently receiving other Complementary Health treatments?
If yes, which ones _____

Do you or have you ever suffered from seizures of any sort?   Yes____   No ____
If yes, please elaborate _____

Are you OK with being touched "appropriately" during a Reiki session or would you prefer not to be touched at all?

                Touch is OK _____   Prefer not to be touched ____

■ **Inappropriate touch of any kind by the Reiki practitioner or the client is a breach of the Reiki Code of Ethics.**

What bothers you about reiki, do you have any concerns, and how does your culture interact with this?
                                        Yes _____   No _____

Insurance

The reader may be wondering why on earth would you need to have Professional Malpractice and General Liability insurance? It shows the practitioner is professional and wants to be taken seriously as having a proper business, also in the event something does happen you are protected.

Preventative Health Services Group in Toronto, ON is a carrier who is familiar with CAM therapies. This policy is part of

Premier Marine – Health & Wellness Liability division. The current level of coverage provides $2,000,000 for liability and $2,000,000 for malpractice.

This policy is only available to Canadian residents. The International Association for Reiki Professionals has U.S. and Canadian sources for insurance.

In researching for insurance, policy prices and coverage can varied widely, the author strongly encourages you to research what is available and ask other practitioners whom they use.

A good starting point would be to connect with different professional organizations like massage, reflexology, and acupuncture and ask their recommendations.

Your car or home insurance provider may cost more and provide less coverage.

Professional Organization

When a practitioner joins an association, (self-regulating body) you can take comfort in knowing others support you. Joining a professional organization helps you the practitioner look professional – adds to your credibility as you are agreeing to certain guidelines and ethical principles. In a sense you and your client are protected, there is a common playing field where you both know what is expected. This group can be a liaison between your chosen field and legislating levels of government.

As a Reiki Practitioner and Teacher, I have joined The Canadian Reiki Association (CRA). This association has changed over the years from a group of people who were interested in promoting, and providing support to Reiki practitioners, to currently working on a set of minimum standards that the various styles of Reiki can live by. This work has included having members document and log client hours for certification with the CRA; all members signing the Code of Ethics and Disciplinary Action forms, and providing advocacy work on its members behalf when local municipal governments are making by-law decisions regarding licensing holistic practitioners. (i.e.: TORONTO MUNICIPAL CODE § 545-158 LICENSING 545-166 **2005 - 12 – 07** ARTICLE XI)

The Association holds yearly conferences, which alternate between Eastern and Western Canada. They can list you on its website and you can subscribe to a quarterly newsletter. For more information go to www.reiki.ca

Some other Reiki Associations (listed in **alphabetical order only**, no ranking has been applied)
Association of Light Touch Therapists:
http://www.altt.org /index.htm
Association of Usui Reiki Healers: http://usuireikihealers.co.uk
Australian Reiki Connection:
http://www.australianreikiconnection.com.au
British Complementary Medicine Association -
http://www.bcma.co.uk/index.html
Council of Australian Reiki Organizations:
http://www.caro.org.au
International Association of Reiki Professionals:
http://www.iarp.org/
International Centre for Reiki Training: William Rand -
http://www.reiki.org/
International House of Reiki: Frans and Bronwen Stiene: -
http://www.reiki.net.au/
International Reiki Association:
http://www.internationalreikiassociation.com
Reiki Australia: http://www.reikiaustralia.com.au
Reiki Healers and Teachers Society:
http://reikihealersandteachers.net
The Reiki Alliance: Phyllis Furumoto: -

http://www.reikialliance.com/
The Reiki Association: http://www.reikiassociation.org.uk
UK Reiki Federation: http://reikifed.co.uk

Like all things, check the associations referenced here and the others that are out in the market place. See if you are in agreement with an associations' mission statement and policies. Contact some of the members and see if the association is organized and supportive. If so, join, if not go the next one on the list.

Bookkeeping

As a small business owner the practitioner would register their business with the Provincial Government. Depending on the products and services provided it would dictate whether or not you would have to collect tax on anything. At the moment in Ontario, holistic practitioners do not have to charge Provincial Sales tax (PST) on our services. This may be changing in the near future as the Provincial government is considering harmonizing (July 2010) the Federal Goods and Service tax (GST) with the PST.

In Canada practitioners can also register their business for a GST number, just remember if you charge GST on a product or service you have to remit that money to the Government, you cannot keep it for yourself.

Once again check with your accountant regarding what taxes are applicable for the services you offer.

Having a practice necessitates the importance of having and maintaining bookkeeping or accounting system when money exchanges hands. Whether it means you learning how to use a computer software program like Quick books or having someone do your "books" for you. In the end you the practitioner are responsible for the cash that flows through your practice.

Your accountant or bookkeeper will assist you in knowing what receipts to keep and what to discard. Remember to keep a mileage log if applicable.

Clients may want a receipt for their records, decide if you want to use a generic receipt book or provide one with your business letterhead.

Personal Hygiene

Reasons for good hygiene:

Looking professional also involves acting professional.

You never get another chance at a first impression.

You are your best calling card — referrals may be your future
   clients.

Clothes:

We would not want our doctors, lawyers, dentists or chiro-practors showing up to work with ripped jeans or comfy sweats. Wear casual dress: nice trousers, comfortable shoes, casual dress shirts, polo or even ones with your business name on. As we are not part of conventional medicine our mode of dress should be anything but medical, for example, no lab coats/smocks, no scrubs. We wouldn't want our clients to have an anxiety attack because our clothes remind them of a traumatic experience in the hospital.

The institutions that regulate massage therapists have guidelines as to what is appropriate for them to wear; the recommendations are easy for Reiki practitioners to follow also.

Denim (jeans/skirts), short-socks, tank/halter tops, mini-skirts, hats or bare midriff/bare shoulders attire are not permitted.[21] This one is easy to remember – it's the three B's: No boobs, bellies or butts.

Grooming:

If you have been running around doing errands before seeing your client, take a moment to make sure your body still smells fresh. Wash the sweat off, and re-apply deodorant if necessary.

Trim and file long fingernails.

Don't get caught with food in-between your teeth, after wolfing down lunch or having that morning bagel. Have a spare toothbrush and paste.

Tie back unruly, wild and crazy hair. If necessary get a haircut, keep the receipt and add it to your accounting expenses.

Be mindful of cologne and perfumes. Some clients have chemical sensitivities that will make them ill if you go crazy with your favourite personal body spray.

Jewelry:

Remove dangling pendants as they could strike your client.

Remove big clunky rings, as your client may not appreciate lying on this hard metal/stone object. The same could be said for bracelets.

Be mindful of any piercings you or your client may have, as getting caught in your client's clothes or blankets could be awkward.

Personal Safety

Clinic or Workspace hygiene

General housekeeping – get rid of the dust bunnies and dirty fingerprints

Use clean linen for each client

Take care of plants – trim if required

Maintain a supply of clean glasses for clients' use

Providing a refreshing drink of water after a reiki session is a good way to revitalize a sleepy client

Being Mindful

If your client arrives and appears to be under the weather (illness), it is your call if you take the risk and work on them or gently suggest that while reiki might assist them in getting better faster, you would prefer if they did their convalescing at home. If your client chooses to go home ask if they would like to be placed on your healing list.

The microscopic germs this client is carrying may not infect you but could infect your next client.

Pathogenic diseases are caused by the presence of one or more pathogenic agent in the body, including viruses, bacteria, fungi, protozoa, multicellular parasites and aberrant proteins known as prions. They damage the hosts; pathogens can include both plants and animals.

The transmission of infectious disease may occur through infected individuals by water, food, airborne inhalation, or though vector borne spread.[22]

Non-pathogenic diseases: are not caused by microbial, bacterial, viral, fungal or parasites. (i.e.: heart disease, menopause, acid reflux.)

What are the routes of exposure?
Pathogens can enter the body through four primary routes:

Inhalation
Contact with blood or other body fluids
Ingestion
Fecal-oral
An intermediate carrier (such as a tick)[23]

What is an airborne disease?
Airborne diseases are spread when droplets of pathogens are expelled into the air due to coughing, sneezing or talking. Airborne diseases of concern to emergency responders

(Emergency response personnel) include:

Meningitis
Chicken pox
Tuberculosis (TB)
Influenza

Many of these diseases require prolonged exposure for infection to occur, posing only minimal threat to emergency responders. However, there are preventive measures, such as wearing masks or maximizing ventilation, that help reduce these risks.[24]

Blood Borne Disease: is defined as any microbiologic agent capable of being transmitted via contact with the blood of an infected individual. Most notably, this includes the human immunodeficiency virus (HIV), hepatititis B virus (HBV), and hepatitis C virus (HCV).
Transmission of Blood Borne Disease may occur if blood or certain body fluids contact tissue under skin (percutaneous injury), non-intact skin or mucous membranes.[25]

Exposure to bloodborne pathogens can occur through many mechanisms: needle sticks, being splashed with blood or body fluids on the mucous membranes (the mouth, eyes, and nose), even in some cases human bites (although the risk of transmission via human bites is extremely low). However, contact with bloodborne pathogens falls into two main categories:

Direct – via an open lesion on the skin or mucous membrane
Indirect – via punctures by contaminated sharps or needles

Bloodborne pathogens enter the body through:

Blood

Other potentially infectious materials (OPIMs), such as:
Body fluids
Amniotic fluid
Semen
Vaginal fluids

Common bloodborne diseases of which first responders (Emergency response personnel) need to be aware include:

Hepatitis B
Hepatitis C
Hepatitis D
AIDS (Acquired Immunodeficiency Syndrome)[26]

What are the modes of transmission?

Exposure occurs through either direct or indirect contact.

Direct transmission occurs when a pathogen an agent that causes disease, esp. a living microorganism such as a bacterium or fungus. Is transmitted directly from an infected individual to you. For example, you could become infected with HBV if you had an open wound that came into contact with a patient's HBV infected blood.

Indirect transmission occurs when an inanimate object serves as a temporary reservoir for the infectious agent. For example, you could become infected with HBV if you come into contact with equipment that has dried infectious blood on it.

It is important to note that many diseases do not manifest themselves immediately. Therefore, it can often be difficult to track the source of an exposure.

Many of the symptoms of some diseases can be quite similar to the flu. Therefore, if flu-like symptoms do not subside in a normal amount of time with normal treatment methods, you may need to have blood tests performed to rule out other possible causes.[27]

Hepatitis A is an acute liver disease caused by the hepatitis A virus (HAV), lasting from a few weeks to several months. It does not lead to chronic infection.

Transmission: Ingestion of fecal matter, even in microscopic amounts, from close person-to-person contact or ingestion of contaminated food or drinks.

Vaccination: Hepatitis A vaccination is recommended for all children starting at age 1 year, travelers to certain countries, and others at risk.

This disease can be associated with fecal contamination of water or food and can be spread person-to-person through poor sanitary habits and the intake of uncooked food or unclean water.

This illness is most commonly seen among children and young adults, but can be most damaging in older adults. Outbreaks are not uncommon at camps or military posts. This is the most common type of viral hepatitis, it can be a problem for fire fighters, especially if their meals are prepared by an infected person or they are infected by contaminated materials at a fire, hazardous materials incident, USAR, or SCUBA incident.[28]

Hepatitis B is a liver disease caused by the hepatitis B virus (HBV). It ranges in severity from a mild illness, lasting a few weeks (acute), to a serious long-term (chronic) illness that can lead to liver disease or liver cancer.

Transmission: Contact with infectious blood, semen, and other body fluids from having sex with an infected person, sharing contaminated needles to inject drugs, or from an infected mother to her newborn.

Vaccination: Hepatitis B vaccination is recommended for all infants, older children and adolescents who were not vaccinated previously, and adults at risk for HBV infection.

Blood infected with the hepatitis B virus is much more infectious than HIV infected blood, and the proportion of the United States population infected with hepatitis B is much higher than the proportion infected with HIV.[29]

Hepatitis C is a liver disease caused by the hepatitis C virus (HCV). HCV infection sometimes results in an acute illness, but most often becomes a chronic condition that can lead to cirrhosis of the liver and liver cancer.

Transmission: Contact with the blood of an infected person, primarily through sharing contaminated needles to inject drugs.

Vaccination: There is no vaccine for hepatitis C.

Hepatitis C is a virus that causes liver disease. HCV is spread by contact with the blood of an infected person. HCV is this country's most common blood borne disease, infecting at least 2 out of every 100 people.

Hepatitis C was formerly known as "non-A, non-B hepatitis" and is currently considered to be a more serious threat to fire fighters, paramedics, and EMTs than the hepatitis B virus. According to the Centers for Disease Control (CDC), hepatitis C is the most common chronic blood borne infection in the United States.[30]

Hepatitis D is a serious liver disease caused by the hepatitis D virus (HDV) and relies on HBV to replicate. It is uncommon in the United States.

Transmission: Contact with infectious blood, similar to how HBV is spread.

Vaccination: There is no vaccine for hepatitis D.

Hepatitis E is a serious liver disease caused by the hepatitis E virus (HEV) that usually results in an acute infection. It does not lead to a chronic infection. While rare in the United States, hepatitis E is common in many parts of the world.

Transmission: Ingestion of fecal matter, even in microscopic amounts; outbreaks are usually associated with contaminated water supply in countries with poor sanitation.

Vaccination: There is currently no FDA-approved vaccine for hepatitis E.[31]

HIV

HIV stands for human immunodeficiency virus. This is the virus that causes AIDS.

HIV is a virus of the type known as retroviruses. These viruses infect certain cells in the body, incorporating their viral genetic material into the cell's own DNA. The body's cells then begin to produce the virus, and in the process, may themselves be killed. In the case of HIV, this virus infects only selected cells in the body, of which the most important are certain infection-fighting white blood cells known as lymphocytes, specifically those lymphocytes known as "helper cells" (which can be identified because they carry a marker called "CD4"). HIV can also infect certain cells in the nervous system.[32] [CD4 cells are also known as T cells]

AIDS

AIDS stands for acquired immunodeficiency syndrome. AIDS is the final stage of HIV infection. It can take years for a person infected with HIV, even without treatment, to reach this stage. Having AIDS means that the virus has weakened the immune system to the point at which the body has a difficult time fighting infection. When someone has one or more specific infections, certain cancers, or a very low number of T cells, he or she is considered to have AIDS.[33]

Viral infectious diseases

AIDS

AIDS Related Complex

Chickenpox (Varicella)

Common cold

Cytomegalovirus Infection

Colorado tick fever

Dengue fever

Ebola hemorrhagic fever

Hand, foot and mouth disease

Hepatitis

Herpes simplex

Herpes zoster

HPV

Influenza (Flu)

Lassa fever

Measles

Marburg hemorrhagic fever

Infectious mononucleosis

Mumps

Norovirus

Poliomyelitis

Progressive multifocal leukencephalopathy

Rabies

Rubella

SARS

Smallpox (Variola)

Viral encephalitis
Viral gastroenteritis
Viral meningitis
Viral pneumonia
West Nile disease
Yellow fever

Parasitic infectious diseases

African trypanosomiasis
Amebiasis
Ascariasis
Babesiosis
Chagas Disease
Clonorchiasis
Cryptosporidiosis
Cysticercosis
Diphyllobothriasis
Dracunculiasis
Echinococcosis
Enterobiasis
Fascioliasis
Fasciolopsiasis
Filariasis
Free-living amebic infection
Giardiasis
Gnathostomiasis
Hymenolepiasis
Isosporiasis
Kala-azar
Leishmaniasis
Malaria
Metagonimiasis
Myiasis
Onchocerciasis

Pediculosis

Pinworm Infection

Scabies

Schistosomiasis

Taeniasis

Toxocariasis

Toxoplasmosis

Trichinellosis

Trichinosis

Trichuriasis

Trichomoniasis

Trypanosomiasis

Prion infectious diseases

Alpers' disease

Fatal Familial Insomnia

Gerstmann-Sträussler-Scheinker syndrome

Kuru – Variant Creutzfeldt-Jakob disease;

q fever,

Mycoses Aspergillosis Aspergillosis,

Allergic   Bronchopulmonary   Neuroaspergillosis
    Blastomycosis Candidiasis Candidiasis,

Chronic Mucocutaneous Candidiasis, Cutaneous Candidiasis,
Oral Candidiasis,

Vulvovaginal Central Nervous System Fungal Infections
    Meningitis,

Fungal + Coccidioidomycosis Cryptococcosis Meningitis,

Cryptococcal Dermatomycoses Blastomycosis Candidiasis,
Chronic Mucocutaneous Candidiasis,

Cutaneous   Chromoblastomycosis   Maduromycosis
    Paracoccidioidomycosis Sporotrichosis Tinea + Tinea
    Versicolor Eye Infections,

Fungal Uveitis, Suppurative + Fungemia Geotrichosis
    Histoplasmosis Lung Diseases,

Fungal Aspergillosis,

Allergic Bronchopulmonary Pneumonia,

Pneumocystis Microsporidiosis Encephalitozoonosis Paracoccidioidomycosis Piedra Pneumocystis Infections Pneumonia,

Pneumocystis Rhinosporidiosis Zygomycosis Mucormycosis

Bacterial infectious diseases

Lyme Disease

Osteomylitis

Meningitis

Celulitis

Syphilis [34]

In the Appendix is a list of pathogenic microbes and infectious diseases that have been discovered between the years 1973 to 1995.

Chapter Review:

Modern medicine is starting to take CAM therapies seriously and incorporating it into their working paradigms. As we are moving into what you would call Integrative Medicine it is important for all players, allopathic and holistic practitioners to begin a dialogue of sharing.

Decide if you are going to be a private practitioner who works out of their home.

Or a practitioner who is going more public by either working out of a home office or having a clinic space.

Have you joined or do you need to join a professional organization?

Have you got insurance or will you need insurance?

Do you need business cards and other promotional literature?

Will you have your clients fill out Consent and Release forms?

Is your Reiki room outfitted with everything you need?

[linen, pillows, music, tissues, glasses, water, etc.]

Do you need to be sensitive to client having challenges to chemical fragrances?

[perfumes, body sprays, fabric softeners, febreze, incense, perfumed candles]

Keep in mind your personal safety, whether it's accepting a new client or working on someone with an illness.

In the event you do get sick and are not able to see your clients form partnerships with other like minded practitioners, so they can help you and your clients out when your stuck.

Always look professional; you never get a second chance.

Chapter 5

Anatomy and Physiology

Depending on the modality learned, there may be a lot of anatomy and physiology learned or there may be none.

For instance, Registered Massage therapists are required to have detailed knowledge on how the body functions. Acupuncture and Acupressure practitioners are also taught this knowledge and the concept of meridians.

Some Energy Medicine modalities like Reiki do not require the practitioner to know this.

The founder of Reiki Mikao Usui is said to have written a book called Reiki Ryoho Hikkei. For now the following quote is from a Q & A about Reiki written in 1922.

Q: *Does the Usui Reiki Ryoho use medications? And are there any kind of side effects?*

A: It uses neither medications nor instruments. It uses only looking, blowing, stroking, (light) tapping, and touching (of the afflicted parts of the body). This is what heals diseases.

Q: *Does a person need medical knowledge in order to use the Usui Reiki Ryoho?*

A: Our ryoho (healing method) is a spiritual method that goes beyond medical science. It therefore is not based upon it.

When you either look at, blow on, touch, or stroke the afflicted part of the body, you will achieve the desired goal. For example, you touch the head when you want to treat the brain, the abdomen when you want to treat the abdomen, and the eyes for the eyes. You take neither bitter medicine nor use hot moxibustion (Chinese moxa herb), and you will be healthy again within a short time. This is why this reiho (spiritual method) is our original creation.

Q: *How do renowned physicians see it (the Usui Reiki Ryoho)?*

A: The educated authorities in this field appear (in the evaluation of the Usui Reiki Ryoho) to be very fair. (These days) well-known European physicians are very critical toward the (stubborn) prescription of medications. As an aside, Dr. Sen Nagai from the Medical Teikoku University said: " We physicians know how to diagnose an illness, record it empirically and understand it, but we do not know how to treat it."

(Another physician) Dr. Kondo said:" It is very arrogant to say that medicine has made tremendous progress since modern medicine neglects the spiritual equilibrium (of the patient). This is its greatest disadvantage." Doctor Sakae Hara said: "It is an impertinence to treat a human being, who possesses spiritual wisdom, like an animal. I believe that we can reckon with a great revolution in the field of therapy in the future."

Dr. Rokura Kuga said: "it is a fact that non-physicians (therapists) have carried out a series of therapies such as psychotherapy with a high degree of success that has not even been achieved by medical faculties because these therapies include the character, the personal symptoms of the patient, and many different (healing) methods in their treatment.

If they (as physicians associated with the medical faculty) would blindly reject therapists and psychotherapists (who are not associated) and attempt to impede them in their work, this would be very narrow-minded."[1]

Physicians and pharmacists often understand this and come to be initiated (by me, by us into Reiki).[1]

The above explanation is helpful in explaining why Reiki practitioners do not go to medical school prior to learning Reiki.

However, the medical community feels that this knowledge would lend credibility to our practice and provide a basis for productive dialogue.

It is at this point some basic medical terminology is in order. Knowing this language will be a helpful point of reference for future note taking, understanding your client's condition and in communication with other support staff.

Our scope of practice is to provide Reiki to our clients, however in order to provide the best possible care we need to familiarize ourselves with our client's condition so that we protect ourselves from pathogenic agents, as well as know what signs and symptoms to look for if and when the client's condition changes.

Basic Terms

Note:

The information presented will not give you any expertise in diagnosing any ailments; please do not attempt to do so unless you are licensed to practice medicine.

Anatomy – is the science of body (plants and animals) structures and their inter-relationships.

Physiology – is the study of mechanical, physical and biochemical properties of living organisms. Physiology incorporates a significant amount of anatomy.

Homeostasis – the tendency towards a relatively stable equilibrium between interdependent elements, esp. as maintained by physiological processes.

Stasis – a state of inactivity or equilibrium.

This section is a review of the important terminology that we will be looking at in a future course.

Our reference is the book "Mastering Healthcare Terminology" by Betsy J. Shiland. Published by Mosby Inc., an affiliate of Elsevier Inc. ISBN: 978-0-323-05506-2

Chapter 1
Root of Healthcare Terms
Key word terms – prefixes, suffixes and combining forms
Abbreviations and symbols

Chapter 2
Body Structure and Directional Terminology
Organization of the Human Body
Anatomic Position and Surface anatomy
Positional and Directional Terms
Planes of the body
Abdominopelvic Regions
Abdominopelvic Quadrants

Chapter 3
Musculoskelatal System
Functions of the Musculoskeletal system
Anatomy and Physiology
Pathology
Diagnostic Procedures
Therapeutic Interventions
Pharmacology
Abbreviations

Chapter 4
Integumentary System
Functions of the Integumentary System
Anatomy and Physiology
Pathology
Diagnostic Procedures
Therapeutic Interventions
Pharmacology
Abbreviations

Chapter 5
Gastrointestinal System

Functions of the Gastrointestinal System

Anatomy and Physiology

Pathology

Diagnostic Procedures

Therapeutic Interventions

Pharmacology

Abbreviations

Chapter 6
Urinary System

Functions of the Urinary System

Anatomy and Physiology

Pathology

Diagnostic Procedures

Therapeutic Interventions

Pharmacology

Abbreviations

Chapter 7 and 8
Male and Female Reproductive Systems

Functions of the Reproductive System

Anatomy and Physiology

Pathology

Diagnostic Procedures

Therapeutic Interventions

Pharmacology

Abbreviations

Chapter 9
Blood, Lymphatic and Immune Systems

Functions of the Blood, Lymphatic & Immune Systems
Anatomy and Physiology
Pathology
Diagnostic Procedures
Therapeutic Interventions
Pharmacology
Abbreviations

Chapter 10)
Cardiovascular System

Functions of the Cardiovascular System
Anatomy and Physiology
Pathology
Diagnostic Procedures
Therapeutic Interventions
Pharmacology
Abbreviations

Chapter 11
Respiratory System

Functions of the Respiratory System
Anatomy and Physiology
Pathology
Diagnostic Procedures
Therapeutic Interventions
Pharmacology
Abbreviations

Chapter 12
Nervous System

Functions of the Nervous System
Anatomy and Physiology

Pathology
Diagnostic Procedures
Therapeutic Interventions
Pharmacology
Abbreviations

Chapter 13
Mental and Behavioral Health

Functions of the Mental and Behavioral Health
Pathology
Diagnostic Procedures
Therapeutic Interventions
Pharmacology
Abbreviations

Chapter 14
Special Senses: Eye and Ear

Functions of the Eye and Ear
Anatomy and Physiology
Pathology
Diagnostic Procedures
Therapeutic Interventions
Pharmacology
Abbreviations

Chapter 15 Endocrine System

Functions of the Endocrine System
Anatomy and Physiology
Pathology
Diagnostic Procedures
Therapeutic Interventions
Pharmacology
Abbreviations

Chapter 16
Oncology

Anatomy can be an interesting subject to learn however don't be blindsided by what your hands may be telling you. On occasion what you are feeling is the end result or referral pain from the original source. Like a good investigator uncover every stone and follow all leads.

Note:
The next two pages of diagrams are to assist non-medical students in gaining perspective where certain organs are located in the human body.

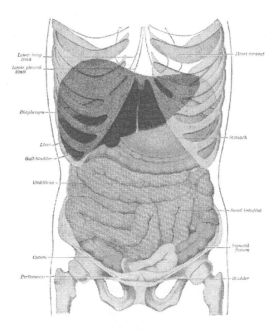

Topography of thoracic and abdominal viscera.

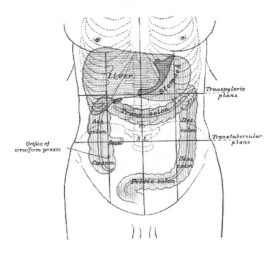

Front of abdomen, showing surface markings for liver, stomach, and great intestine.

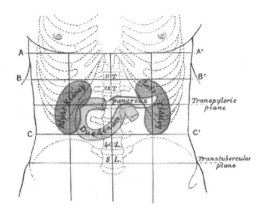

Front of abdomen, showing surface markings for duodenum, pancreas, and kidneys. *A A'*. Plane through joint between body and xiphoid process of sternum. *B B'*. Plane midway between *A A'* and transpyloric plane. *C C'*. Plane midway between transpyloric and transtubercular planes.

Chapter Review:

During the age in which Reiki was established, it was not necessary for students to know modern anatomical positions. However, in an effort to form a meaningful partnership with other members of the healthcare team, it is wise to have a basic knowledge of anatomy and physiology.

The medical terminology book will assist students in understanding some of the apparent complicated language that exists within the modern allopathic medical system. Each chapter has its own exercises and you are responsible for learning the content.

Chapter 6

Creating that Therapeutic Relationship with Clients and Caregivers

The contents of this section have a Reiki focus as that is the modality the author practices. However, the subject matter is easily changeable to any modality: Homeopathy, Naturopathy, Acupuncture, Traditional Chinese Medicine, Reflexology, Bowen Technique, Aromatherapists, Music and Art therapists, etc.

When discussing Reiki with your client, their caregivers or guardians, there are many things we as practitioners need to share, in addition to the three C's: Code of Conduct, Consent and Confidentiality and remember Cultural Competency. [Chapter 4]

The Reiki you offer in your clinic is no different than when you offer it to someone in a hospital, palliative or hospice care setting.

There are some similarities like having the client fill in the Consent and Release form, maintaining confidentiality, and conducting yourself in a professional manner. However there are some mechanical differences when offering Reiki in an institutional location.

This chapter covers the consultation process, appropriate client care, keeping the lines of communication open between clients and possibly a health care team and therapeutic boundaries.

When accepting a new client it is always good to go through an interview type process to see if there is a "good fit" or easy rapport. The boundaries you establish now will go a long way in preventing any miscommunication or misunderstandings later on.

Don't be surprised if your client/caregiver/guardian asks you questions too. This is a good thing as they are expressing interest in the service you're providing as well as ensuring that their loved one or themselves are getting the highest quality care.

They may ask you about your Reiki training, how long you have been doing Reiki, have you had any other clients, or even what kind of experience have you had with this kind of illness.

At this time ask your potential client or caregivers/guardians any of your questions so that both of you are clear on what is expected.

For instance: Ask if there would be any problem giving the potential client a drink of water once the Reiki session is over. This question is important just in case the volume of fluids needs to be measured, everyone involved needs to know. However if your client or the caregiver/guardian asks you to administer any medication, explain to whoever is asking that legally you are not qualified to do so. Remember only do what you are qualified for; if your scope of practice is only Reiki then do only Reiki. If your scope of practice includes being a personal support worker (PSW), occupational therapist (OT), registered nurse (RN), etc., then discuss with the client and caregiver/guardian what steps you would take if an emergency situation arose.

In the above instance, if you are providing Reiki to a client and an emergency does arise, what do you do and whom should you call? Discuss this scenario with the caregiver or guardian, so you are clear about whom to contact. Do you call the caregiver/guardian, is there a do not resuscitate order (DNR) or emergency - 911?

Let's say the big day has arrived and you are introduced to your new client and their caregiver.

Both you and your client may be nervous, but soon those initial awkward moments will be forgotten as your warm, caring and sincere approach puts everyone at ease.

During volunteer training for Hospice, we were counselled in the fine art of communication.

As the communication section is quite concise this is a direct quote from the manual.[1]

Techniques that help communication:

Giving recognition:
Good morning, Mr. Smith
You've written some letters today.
I notice you've chosen your favourite music for today.

Giving information:
My name is …
I'm here because
I'll be taking you to the …

Giving broad openings:
How do you feel? (Today)
Is there something you'd like to talk about?
Where would you like to begin?

Accepting:
I understand…
I agree…
I hadn't thought of that…

Using silence:
Yes, Uh-huh, Hummm, nodding.

Offering general leads:
Go on and then?
Tell me about it?

Placing the event in time:
What seemed to lead up to ...?
or in sequence:
Was this before or after...?
When did this happen...?

Making observations:
Are you uncomfortable when you ...?
I notice you are biting your lips.

Encouraging description:
Tell me when you began to feel anxious.
How would you describe your pain?

Restating:
Client: I seem to hear the clock strike every hour during the night.
Volunteer: You have difficulty sleeping?

Note: When using restating, do not overdo the obvious. Only restate complex statements or those that seem to have an unspoken message behind them.

Reflecting:
Client: Do you think I should tell the doctor?
Volunteer: Do **you** think you should?

Note: In this case there seems to be an underlying emotion. Does the client sound frustrated, or excited?

Attempting to translate feelings:
Client: I can't talk to you or to anyone. It's a waste of time.
Volunteer: Do you feel no one understands?

Client: I'm way out in the ocean.

Volunteer: Do you mean you feel abandoned?

Seeking clarification:
I'm not sure that I follow.
What would you say is the main point of what you said?
May I tell you what I think you said?

Focusing:
This point seems worth looking at more closely,

Encouraging a plan of action:
Next time this family problem comes up, what might you do to handle it?
What could you do to let your anger out harmlessly?

Offering self:
I'll sit with you a while.
I'm interested in making you comfortable.
Perhaps you and I can discover what might reduce your anxiety.

Summary:
Why do you think that?
Why do you feel this way?
What made you do that?

Techniques that Block Communication:

Offering false reassurance:
I wouldn't worry about ...
Everything will be all right.
You're coming along fine.

Expressing judgement:
That's good. I'm glad that you...

That's bad. I'd rather you wouldn't...

Advising:
I think you should...
Why don't you ...

Disagreeing:
I definitely disagree with...
I don't believe that.
Client: I'm nothing.
Volunteer: Of course you're something.
Everybody is somebody.

Defending:
No one here would lie to you.
But Mrs. B. is a very capable caregiver.

Making stereotyped comments:
It's for your own good.
Keep your chin up.
Just listen to your doctor ... he knows

Introducing an unrelated topic:
Client: I'd like to die.
Volunteer: Did you have any visitors today?

Using jargon:
Volunteer: I hear you saying that...

Why would:
Putting someone on the spot

Patronizing:
Don't talk down to the client

Being overly chatty:
Constantly talking

Butting in:
Constantly interrupting

Non-Verbal Communication

Note: Seventy-five percent of communication is non-verbal. During personal contact, as you visit a client, the following will lay a foundation for a trusting, open relationship. Hopefully this will be a relationship where you can employ our skills to help the client overcome personal obstacles and gain strength and insight into him/herself.

Body Language

Body language involves: posture, speed (talking and walking), rhythm, gestures (fidgeting, rubbing hands, tapping foot, shrugging, squinting), physical appearance (grooming and wearing apparel).

Body language can reflect mood, mask feelings, contradict verbal message, transmit anxiety.

We tend to mirror those we speak to (e.g. adapt to their rhythm, scratch if they scratch).

Always remember that different nationalities may use different non-verbal cues.

A relaxed body will generally convey the best messages.

Personal Space

Personal space generally refers to the distance one stands from another during conversation.

There are definite cultural differences in personal space.

Intrusion into another's personal space may strip the other person of dignity, whereas standing at too great a distance may communicate lack of genuine concern or physical repulsion.

Generally there should be about 1.5 to 3 feet (46 cm to 91 cm) between visitor and client during conversation.

It helps to remove physical obstacles, such as a bedside table, which may separate you.

Eye and Facial Expressions

Eye and facial expressions are the most readable non-verbal communication.

Facial expressions signal emotions (e.g. smile, frown, surprise, anger, wince, boredom).

Eye contact is essential to communicate sincerity and interest.

Looking away from a person may suggest avoidance, insecurity, and distraction.

It takes a conscious effort to look into a person's eyes and not just at the person or past him/her.

Eye and facial expressions signal emotions and may unconsciously transmit messages that contradict our words.

The Environment

The environment is often overlooked.

The physical environment can transmit a mood (e.g. overcrowding, dull colours, noisy, soft colours, bright/sunny rooms, pictures on the wall, flowers in sight, carpets on the floor, soft music).

The mood that the environment transmits may be conducive to the healing process.

Our physical presence is also a part of the environment; what we wear may send a message to the client (e.g. reluctance to remove our coat may denote a short hurried visit).

To convey a friendly message, we should sit and talk with a client in a position that is comfortable for the client to view us; we should avoid having our back to a window or bright light, since this will make it difficult for the client to face us.

Talking to the client on the same level of eye contact communicates equality and respect rather than dominance.

Sometimes allowing the client to be the higher person through squatting beside the bed or sitting on a low stool conveys a respect and give the client a sense of dominance seldom experienced in a hospital setting.

Touching

Touching is the act of feeling with the hand or other bodily part.

Touch is the most powerful non-verbal form of communication

Hugs, kisses, stroking actually transmit energy. It has been said that one needs: 4 hugs a day for survival, 8 for maintenance, and 12 for growth.

A hand, gently placed on the client's shoulder will convey caring.

Touching induces relaxation which can relieve anxiety and even lessen pain.

Touch is also a reality orienting technique (e.g. when offering a cold drink to a client, encourage him to feel the coldness of the glass even if he cannot hold the glass by himself; encourage the client to touch clothing and feel the texture, or touch the leaves and petals of a floral bouquet.

When touching, be sure to use decisive strokes, if the touch is tentative, messages of anxiety or dislike are transmitted.

If there is no touching, we communicate a lack of warmth.

However, personality styles and cultural differences may dictate the degree of touching, the visitor must be sensitive to the client's responses, whether positive or negative.

Tone of Voice

Tone of voice is especially important during bereavement calls.

Softness of voice, unhurried responses, a degree of calm interest will convey comfort and concern and transmit an energy to the bereaved person.

In conversation with a client, the visitor's tone of voice may bring comfort and reassurance or spark annoyance and non-compliance.

Always Remember:
A SMILE IS OFTEN THE BEST NON-VERBAL COMMUNI-CATION!

Active Listening Skills

Attentive listening is a highly developed skill that is essential. [for hospice volunteers] It is an active process that requires energy and concentration. It involves attention to the person's total message, both the spoken verbal messages and the non-verbal messages that modify what is spoken. The listener must also be aware of his or her own cultural and ethnic influences (cultural competence) as well as those of the client and/or family member. The listener must make a special effort not to select or listen to solely what he or she wants to hear. Instead, he or she must focus on the other person's needs, rather than his /her own, to get the full picture.

Here are some guidelines for active listening:

Be silent. Silence is more than staying quiet or not interrupting while someone is speaking. Before you start to talk pause to allow the speaker to catch his/her breath or gather his/her thoughts. He/she may want to continue.

If the message is complete, this short break gives you time to form your response and helps you avoid the biggest barrier to listening: listening with your answer running. If you make up a response before the person is finished, you miss the end of the message that often contains the main point.

At the same time, use common sense. Pausing for several seconds may be inappropriate. For example when someone asks for assistance with moving or for a comfort measure.

Remain at eye level. Make certain that you are at eye level with the client. Whether or not you look directly at the client depends on the client's comfort level. Cultural considerations come into play. However, in most cases, looking at the other person while he/she speaks demonstrates your attention and helps keep your mind from wandering.

Sit beside a person at a 45-degree angle, if possible, to allow them to look away from your eye contact if they wish. Try to be the same height as the person. If your client is in bed or sitting down, do not stand over them while you talk.

Display openness. You can communicate openness by your facial expressions and body positions. Uncross your arms. Sit comfortably and informally. Sit beside the person and remove any physical barriers, such as a pile of books. Facing a person directly opposite them may be very intimidating and unsupportive.

Listen without response. This doesn't mean never respond. It means wait. When listening to another person, we often interrupt with our opinions, suggestions, and inappropriate comments.

Watch your non-verbal response, too. A look of "Good grief!" from you can keep the other person from finishing his/her message.

Send acknowledgements. Periodically, it is important to let the speaker know you are still there. Your words or non-verbal gestures of acknowledgement let the speaker know you are interested and that you are with him/her and his/her message. These include "Uh uh," "OK," "Hummm.." and head nods.

These acknowledgements do not imply your agreement. If someone tells you what he/she does not like about you, your head nod doesn't mean you agree. It just indicates that you are listening.

Use physical contact only with permission. Communication through touch can be very effective. However you must ask permission first. It can be as simple as asking the client if you may hold his/her hand or "give them a hug". It is essential to obtain this "consent" from the client and/or family member before touching.

Communicating with Someone in a Coma

Coma is a state of unconsciousness. Touching, shaking or calling cannot rouse a person in a coma. This does not mean that a person in a coma cannot hear and understand your voice or feel your touch. Coma is not always permanent, nor does it mean that death is always near, even in the terminally ill. Some people will slip in and out of coma; some will suddenly just wake up. Whatever the cause or duration of the coma, it must not keep you from communicating with the person.

When someone we know or love goes into a coma, it triggers feelings in us. We can feel hurt, cut off, helpless, depressed, confused, angry, grief-stricken. The person has changed and the life force and personality have been turned inward.

To communicate with a person in a coma, you need to become

aware of both your own and the other person's inner feelings and perceptions. You need to look for tiny clues, subtle messages. Changes in breathing pattern, tiny facial changes, changes in relation or rigidity of the person's body are all clues to how he or she is feeling. Once you are aware of these clues you will be able to send and receive messages. Trust your "sixth sense": your intuition, when you are trying to communicate with a person in coma.

Speak normally. Tell him/her what you see and feel. Encourage him/her to feel what he/she is feeling.

Use touch as a way of communicating. Placing your hand on the person's chest and breathing when he/she breathes will help you to tune into the person's inner world. (Telling them that you will be placing your hand on their chest before starting.)

Remember that a coma is an inner experience. Do not try to make the person come out of it. The inner experience is a part of dying and for most people it is a necessary experience.

Be relaxed and calm inside yourself. You do not have to communicate all the time. The person experiencing the coma has less awareness of the external environment.

Remember that your touch, tone of voice, and inner feelings are all perceptible to the person in the coma.

Confidentiality

Confidentiality means "entrusted with secrets". Every [Hospice Palliative Care Volunteer] is required to respect the confidentiality of client and family member information. In addition to protecting the privacy of each client and/or family member, respecting confidentiality is fundamental to providing high quality [hospice palliative] care:

It meets the basic need for privacy and the universal expectation that one's privacy will be respected

It protects the client and family members from public embarrassment or prejudice

It creates an atmosphere of trust in which the dying person and family members are more likely to share information vital to his or her care and support

Privacy is an important factor in client and family satisfaction with care and support

A simple rule for maintaining confidentiality:

Anything you

See

Hear

Read

Observe with your five senses

Already know about the client and family members

Must be kept confidential.

Breaching of confidentiality is a serious breach of ethics [and may result in the termination of a Hospice Palliative Care Volunteer].

Limits to confidentiality

Confidentiality can be breached when there is an unacceptable risk of harm to the individual or someone else, and such circumstances would include:

Certain communicable diseases that must be reported by law to the authorities – this is done by the nurse and/or physician

A medical condition (e.g. mental illness) that may result in personal harm or harm to others

Reasonable suspicion of abuse

Remember, as discussed in the previous section, Confidentiality is also the law.

What we have just covered in communication between a client and caregiver can easily be extended and expanded upon when you are part of a health care team.

Your observation and communication skills are indispensable when interacting with a client and will assist everyone in the health care team stay up to date.

Therefore as part of a health care team, you may be asked to take notes; other times not. You may just take notes only to remind yourself of what transpired the last time you worked with this client. On the occasions when you are asked to make notes they may take on a more formal nature in the structure of a case report (mentioned in Chapter 3) or a S.O.A.P. note.

The basic format for a medical SOAP note:

S Subjective: any information you receive from the patient (history of present illness, past medical history, etc)

O Objective: any data, whether in the form of a physical finding during your exam, or lab results

A Assessment: diagnoses derived from the history and objective data

P Plan: what you intend to do about the diagnoses from your assessment

Sample abbreviations:

ON (overnight), NAD (no acute distress), UOP (urine output), Ms (bowel movements), POD# 3(post-op day 3), lap chole (laparascopic cholecystectomy).[2]

It is not just Allopathic medicine that uses SOAP notes, Chiropractors, Traditional Chinese Medicine practitioners, even Massage and Occupational therapists will use this charting system to record a clients condition. As a member of the healthcare team, Reiki practitioners need to know how to record their subjective observations to share with other members of the team.

Why?[3]

So why do Occupational Therapists - OT's (and others) need to write notes? A few reasons:

Legal/Ethical responsibility: Necessary under COT code of ethics (3.4) (ALL records are officially the property of the Secretary of State – this is a United States website)

Statistics/Audits - used to measure success of intervention & for research

For following progress of colleagues work

The various varieties of notes

So writing clear, concise easy-to-understand but also professional notes is essential - but do we need to write lengthy notes about everything? Well not quite - often notes will get broken down into a number of areas including telephone contact sheets for quick relevant calls, referral forms, assessment forms, reports and discharge summaries. However the large volume of notes that are scrutinised more than any other are the day-to-day client progress notes - the ones detailing actual intervention and the main port of call for any health professional. For all notes the majority of health professionals follow some form of standards for record keeping — directed by either their health authority or/and the overarching professional body. For OT in the UK this can be found in the "Standards for Practice: Occupational Therapy Record Keeping" which outlines the requirements of all records written and kept by an OT.

Some of the commonly used guidelines include that notes should:

be legible & jargon free - check with your department as to the specific shorthand acronyms - some go as far as no acronyms so beware! (even things like TV can be "banned")

be made within 24 hours

be signed and dated by the author

avoid opinion & record only facts observed.

Subjective info should be identified as such show that you are addressing all the identified needs. Don't say you are going to do about a certain need if you can't not be altered, unless the error is crossed out but still readable

not have tipp-ex on them

not have lines with blank spaces on. You should put a straight line across lines to fill them. This is to stop you writing notes at a later date.

not contain a diagnosis made by someone who is not qualified to make one - write the symptoms instead e.g. "Doris has signs & symptoms of xxx. Can medical team please assess"

not record assumptions. for example - you shouldn't state "the patient appeared sad." Unless of course it is justified.

Note that the last two points are tricky. Let's think about the following:

"I went to see Mrs X who is suffering from an acute episode of clinical depression. She appeared low in mood and angry that she wasn't allowed off the ward today"

So how would you write this knowing the previous points? Well classically you would write:

"Meeting with Mrs X. Mrs X appeared low in mood and showed anger towards the OT that she was not allowed off the ward"

Hmm. Well lovely as that is, it's dangerous on a few grounds. Who says she is low in mood? Your view of appearing low in mood may be completely different How did she show "anger"? What did she do? It's much harder to write, but this would be better:

"Meeting with Mrs X. Mrs X reported to feel low and tearful. Discussed with OT how she is angry and confused that she is not allowed off the ward. OT discussed with her the concerns regarding her mental state and sectioning system"

SOAP Note Format

Or what is now commonly called SOAP has its history in the POMR - Problem Orientated Medical Records system (Weed, 1971). This was drawn up to:

improve communication among all those caring for the patient

display the assessment, problems and plans in an organized format to facilitate the care of the patient

use in record review and quality control

There are four commonly used components of SOAP:

S = Subjective (what the client Said - e.g. their reported feelings

O = Objective (what you Observed - e.g. what you did. NB: not your subjective interpretation)

A = Assessment (the Analysis of Subjective & Objective)

P = Plan

In detail:

Subjective

Presents the problems from the patients viewpoint — how he/she may feel. ""Information from other individuals also go here. Relevant info also include:

The reason for the patients visit — often in the patients own words

History of presenting condition/function in chronological age

Symptoms data including severity, location, duration & frequency of symptoms the patient is experiencing

Past medical/social history

Medications being currently taken as well as appetite, diet and allergies

Objective

Records the physical symptoms and includes specific objective statements. Can be gathered from Observation of the patient, Physical Examination, Lab results and X-Rays for example. More than often it consists of what you observe. Note that it is this part that is often scrutinised for accuracy - don't make observations unless they wouldn't be observed the same way as someone else - e.g. X was crying and not X was sad.

Assessment/Analysis

Interpretation of the subjective/objective elements.

Plan

Describes plan for treatment/further sessions and management of the noted issues. Could include referral, phone call or plan to collect more information. Note that some people often use this as objective style plan - a client-centred, specific and measurable plan of intervention by a set time (SMART).

Note that some people will put Objective before Subjective statements - arguing that they are easier to write - it doesn't matter just as long as it's all in there! It's also often wise to put a little line before the SOAP just stating what the note entry is for (e.g. visit, phone call, discharge etc..)

Soap Note		
	Date:	Time:
Client	Name: Age: Address: M or F Phone: Notify: Relation: Phone:	
Subjective		
Objective		
Assessment		
Plan		

Check with the other members of the health care team and inquire if they have noticed any changes in the client.

Is the client's condition improving or declining?

Happier or sad, talkative or quiet, engaging in life or pulling away?

Depending on what is going on with the client and or their caregiver you could further assist them by being aware of what support agencies are available your area. Is it time to get these agencies involved if they have not been used in the past? In this manner you can be an advocate for the client and caregiver.

Do they need extra emotional support?

Do they need a caseworker to assess what they need?

Does the main caregiver need a break?

Is the caregiver starting to show signs of burnout, due to being the sole provider of care?

Do they need help bathing, feeding or moving the client?

As the illness progresses is your client aware of any new treatment options?

Does your client have all the telephone numbers for financial assistance, and palliative care?

The Ontario Ministry of Health and Long-Term Care has set up local Health service centres.

Each local Community Care Access Centre (CCAC) has the resources to assist the client or caregiver with home care, long-term care destinations, and other services in your community.

I would encourage those of you not living in Ontario to contact your Ministry of Health and Long-Term care to see if they have set-up a similar program.

Another resource is the Canadian Hospice Palliative Care Association. (CHPACA)

This is part of CHPACA's working definition:
Hospice palliative care is appropriate for any patient and /or family living with, or at risk of developing, a life-threatening illness due to any diagnosis, with any prognosis, regardless of age, and at any time they have unmet expectations and/or needs, and are prepared to accept care.[4]

When taking your own notes you may develop a short hand that works well for you. However, if sharing this same information with other members of the health care team they may not understand what you have written. In the appendix of the book *Mastering Healthcare Terminology*, by Betsy Shiland has a list of common abbreviations.

Types of Common illnesses:

Cancer
HIV AIDS
Cardiac (heart) disease
Renal (kidney) disease
Hepatic (liver) failure
Pulmonary (lung) disease
Neurological
ALS (Amyotrophic Lateral Sclerosis, Lou Gherigs disease
Multiple Sclerosis
Alzheimer's
Parkinson's

Medline Plus (Online) Medical Encyclopaedia was the source for providing information on the major disorders listed below and the definitions of some common ailments.

Hodgkin's lymphoma: a cancer of lymph tissue found in the lymph nodes, spleen, liver, bone marrow, and other sites.

Non- Hodgkin's lymphoma: cancer of the lymphoid tissue, which includes the lymph nodes, spleen, and other organs of the immune system. There are many different types of non Hodgkin's lymphoma.

Leukemia is a group of bone marrow diseases involving an uncontrolled increase in white blood cells (leukocytes).

Multiple myeloma; Plasma cell dyscrasia; Plasma cell myeloma; Malignant plasmacytoma; Plasmacytoma of bone; is cancer of the plasma cells in bone marrow. Plasma cells help the body's immune system fight disease by producing substances called antibodies. In multiple myeloma, plasma cells grow out of control and form tumors in the bone marrow.

The excess growth of plasma cells interferes with the body's ability to make red blood cells, white blood cells, and platelets. This causes anaemia, which makes a person more likely to get infections and have abnormal bleeding.

As the cancer cells grow in the bone marrow, they can cause pain and destruction of the bones. If the bones in the spine are affected, it can put pressure on the nerves, resulting in numbness or paralysis.

Multiple myeloma mainly affects older adults. A history of radiation therapy raises your risk for this type of cancer.

Angina is a type of chest discomfort caused by poor blood flow through the blood vessels (coronary vessels) of the heart muscle (myocardium).

Arrhythmias are a disorder of the heart rate (pulse) or heart rhythm, such as beating too fast (tachycardia), too slow (bradycardia), or irregularly.

Coronary artery disease (CAD) Arteriosclerotic heart disease, or Coronary heart disease (CHD) is a narrowing of the small blood vessels that supply blood and oxygen to the heart.

Congenital heart disease refers to a problem with the heart's structure and function due to abnormal heart development before birth. Congenital means present at birth.

Heart attack (myocardial infarction) Myocardial infarction; MI; Acute MI; ST-elevation myocardial infarction; non-ST-elevation myocardial infarction A heart attack is when blood vessels that supply blood to the heart are blocked, preventing enough oxygen from getting to the heart. The heart muscle dies or becomes permanently damaged.

Mitral valve prolapse; Barlow syndrome; Floppy mitral valve; Myxomatous mitral valve; Billowing mitral valve; Systolic click-murmur syndrome; Prolapsing mitral leaflet syndrome is a heart problem in which the valve that separates the upper and lower chambers of the left side of the heart does not close properly.

Congestive heart failure (CHF) or Heart failure is a life-threatening condition in which the heart can no longer pump enough blood to the rest of the body.

Chronic kidney failure; Kidney failure - chronic; Renal failure - chronic; Chronic renal insufficiency; Chronic renal failure is a slowly worsening loss of the ability of the kidneys to remove wastes, concentrate urine, and conserve electrolytes.

End-stage renal disease; Renal failure - end stage; Kidney failure - end stage, ESRD is the complete, or almost complete failure of the kidneys to function. The kidneys can no longer remove wastes, concentrate urine, and regulate electrolytes.

Renal artery embolism; Acute renal arterial thrombosis; Renal artery embolism; Acute renal artery occlusion; Embolism - renal artery is an occlusion of the kidney that is a sudden, severe blockage of the artery that supplies blood to the kidney.

Interstitial nephritis; Tubulointerstitial nephritis; Nephritis - interstitial; Acute interstitial (allergic) nephritisis is a kidney disorder in which the spaces between the kidney tubules become swollen (inflamed). The inflammation can affect the kidneys' ability to filter waste.

Reye's syndrome or Reye syndrome is sudden (acute) brain damage (encephalopathy) and liver function problems of unknown cause.

The syndrome has occurred with the use of aspirin to treat chickenpox or the flu in children. However, it has become very uncommon since aspirin is no longer recommended for routine use in children.

Wilson's disease[5] Hepatolenticular degeneration is an inherited disorder in which there is too much copper in the body's tissues. The excess copper damages the liver and nervous system.

Cirrhosis or Liver cirrhosisis caused by chronic liver disease. Common causes of chronic liver disease in the U.S. include: Hepatitis C infection, and long-term alcohol abuse.

Chronic obstructive pulmonary disease (COPD), Chronic obstructive airways disease; Chronic obstructive lung disease; Chronic bronchitis; Emphysema; Bronchitis – chronic is lung disease that makes it difficult to breathe. There are two main forms of COPD:

Chronic bronchitis, which causes long-term swelling and a large amount of mucus in the main airways in the lungs

Emphysema, a lung disease that destroys the air sacs in the lungs Most people with COPD have symptoms of both.

Pulmonary tuberculosis TB; Tuberculosis – pulmonary is a contagious bacterial infection that mainly involves the lungs, but may spread to other organs.

Rheumatoid lung disease or Lung disease - rheumatoid arthritis; Rheumatoid nodules is a group of lung problems related to rheumatoid arthritis. The condition can include fluid in the chest (pleural effusions), scarring (pulmonary fibrosis), lumps (nodules), and high blood pressure in the lungs (pulmonary hypertension).

Amyotrophic Lateral Sclerosis (ALS), Lou Gehrig's disease; Upper and lower motor neuron disease; Motor neuron disease is a disease of the nerve cells in the brain and spinal cord that control voluntary muscle movement. In ALS, nerve cells (neurons) waste away or die, and can no longer send messages to muscles. This eventually leads to muscle weakening, twitching, and an inability to move the arms, legs, and body. The condition slowly gets worse. When the muscles in the chest area stop working, it becomes hard or impossible to breathe on one's own.

Huntington's disease or Huntington chorea is a disorder passed down through families in which nerve cells in the brain waste away, or degenerate.

Muscular dystrophy (MD), Inherited myopathy; Muscular dystrophy is a group of disorders that involve muscle weakness and loss of muscle tissue that get worse over time.

Multiple sclerosis (MS), Demyelinating disease, is an autoimmune disease that affects the brain and spinal cord (central nervous system).

Parkinson's or Paralysis agitans; Shaking palsy is a disorder of the brain that leads to shaking (tremors) and difficulty with walking, movement, and coordination.

Senile dementia/Alzheimer's type (SDAT) Alzheimer's disease (AD), one form of dementia, is a progressive, degenerative brain disease. It affects memory, thinking, and behavior.

Memory impairment is a necessary feature for the diagnosis of this or any type of dementia. Change in one of the following areas must also be present: language, decision-making ability, judgment, attention, and other areas of mental function and personality.

The rate of progression is different for each person. If AD develops rapidly, it is likely to continue to progress rapidly. If it has been slow to progress, it will likely continue on a slow course.

Others:

Fibromyalgia or Fibromyositis; Fibrositis is a common condition characterized by long-term, body-wide pain and tender points in joints, muscles, tendons, and other soft tissues. Fibromyalgia has also been linked to fatigue, morning stiffness, sleep problems, headaches, numbness in hands and feet, depression, and anxiety.
Fibromyalgia can develop on its own or along with other musculoskeletal conditions such as rheumatoid arthritis or lupus.
Chronic Fatigue, CFS; Fatigue - chronic; Immune dysfunction syndrome Chronic fatigue syndrome is a condition of prolonged

and severe tiredness or weariness (fatigue) that is not relieved by rest and is not directly caused by other conditions. To be diagnosed with this condition, your tiredness must be severe enough to decrease your ability to participate in ordinary activities by 50%.

I would strongly recommend going to this website if any of the conditions listed in the categories below are of interest to you.

Cancer is mentioned below
HIV AIDS was discussed in chapter 4

Cardiovascular disorders
Heart disease is any disorder that affects the heart's ability to function normally. Various forms of heart disease include:
Alcoholic cardiomyopathy
Aortic regurgitation
Aortic stenosis
Arrhythmias
Cardiogenic shock
Congenital heart disease
Coronary artery disease (CAD)
Dilated cardiomyopathy
Endocarditis
Heart attack (myocardial infarction)
Heart failure
Heart tumor
Hypertrophic cardiomyopathy
Idiopathic cardiomyopathy
Ischemic cardiomyopathy
Acute mitral regurgitation
Chronic mitral regurgitation
Mitral stenosis
Mitral valve prolapse

Peripartum cardiomyopathy

Pulmonary stenosis

Stable angina

Unstable angina

Tricuspid regurgitation [6]

Renal disorders are diseases of the kidneys.

Urological disorders are diseases of the kidneys/urinary tract.[7]

Kidney disease is any disease or disorder that affects the function of the kidneys. This may include:

Acute kidney failure

Acute nephritic syndrome

Analgesic nephropathy

Atheroembolic renal disease

Chronic kidney failure

Chronic nephritis

Congenital nephrotic syndrome

End-stage renal disease

Goodpasture syndrome

Interstitial nephritis

Kidney cancer

Kidney damage

Kidney infection

Kidney injury

Kidney stones

Lupus nephritis

Membranoproliferative GN I

Membranoproliferative GN II

Membranous nephropathy

Minimal change disease

Necrotizing glomerulonephritis

Nephroblastoma

Nephrocalcinosis

Nephrogenic diabetes insipidus

Nephropathy - IgA

Nephrosis (nephrotic syndrome)

Polycystic kidney disease

Post-streptococcal GN

Reflux nephropathy

Renal artery embolism

Renal artery stenosis

Renal disorders

Renal papillary necrosis

Renal tubular acidosis type I

Renal tubular acidosis type II

Renal underperfusion

Renal vein thrombosis [8]

Hepatic Disorders The term "liver disease" applies to many diseases and disorders that cause the liver to function improperly or cease functioning. Abnormal results of liver function tests often suggest liver disease. See also

Amebic liver abscess

Autoimmune hepatitis

Biliary atresia

Cirrhosis

Coccidioidomycosis; disseminated

Delta agent (Hepatitis D)

Drug-induced cholestasis

Hemochromatosis

Hepatitis A

Hepatitis B

Hepatitis C

Hepatocellular carcinoma

Liver cancer

Liver disease due to alcohol

Primary biliary cirrhosis
Pyogenic liver abscess
Reye's syndrome
Sclerosing cholangitis
Wilson's disease [9]

Pulmonary Disorders Lung disease is any disease or disorder that occurs in the lungs or that causes the lungs to not work properly. There are three main types of lung disease:

Airway diseases — These diseases affect the tubes (airways) that carry oxygen and other gases into and out of the lungs. These diseases cause a narrowing or blockage of the airways. They include asthma, emphysema, and chronic bronchitis. People with airway diseases sometimes describe the feeling as "trying to breathe out through a straw."

Lung tissue diseases — These diseases affect the structure of the lung tissue. Scarring or inflammation of the tissue makes the lungs unable to expand fully ("restrictive lung disease"). It also makes the lungs less capable of taking up oxygen (oxygenation) and releasing carbon dioxide. Pulmonary fibrosis and sarcoidosis are examples of lung tissue diseases. People sometimes describe the feeling as "wearing a too-tight sweater or vest" that won't allow them to take a deep breath.

Pulmonary circulation diseases — These diseases affect the blood vessels in the lungs. They are caused by clotting, scarring, or inflammation of the blood vessels. They affect the ability of the lungs to take up oxygen and to release carbon dioxide. These diseases may also affect heart function.

Most lung diseases actually involve a combination of these categories.

The most common lung diseases include:
Asthma
Chronic bronchitis

COPD (chronic obstructive pulmonary disease)
Emphysema
Pulmonary fibrosis
Sarcoidosis

Other lung diseases include:
Asbestosis
Aspergilloma
Aspergillosis
Aspergillosis - acute invasive
Atelectasis
Eosinophilic pneumonia
Lung cancer
Metastatic lung cancer
Necrotizing pneumonia
Pleural effusion
Pneumoconiosis
Pneumocystosis
Pneumonia
Pneumonia in immunodeficient patient
Pneumothorax
Pulmonary actinomycosis
Pulmonary alveolar proteinosis
Pulmonary anthrax
Pulmonary arteriovenous malformation
Pulmonary edema
Pulmonary embolus
Pulmonary histiocytosis X (eosinophilic granuloma)
Pulmonary hypertension
Pulmonary nocardiosis
Pulmonary tuberculosis
Pulmonary veno-occlusive disease
Rheumatoid lung disease [10]

Neurologic diseases are disorders of the brain, spinal cord and nerves throughout your body. Together they control all the workings of the body. When something goes wrong with a part of your nervous system, you can have trouble moving, speaking, swallowing, breathing or learning. You can also have problems with your memory, senses or mood.

There are more than 600 neurologic diseases. Major types include:

Diseases caused by faulty genes, such as Huntington's disease and muscular dystrophy

Problems with the way the nervous system develops, such as spina bifida

Degenerative diseases, where nerve cells are damaged or die, such as Parkinson's disease and Alzheimer's disease

Diseases of the blood vessels that supply the brain, such as stroke

Injuries to the spinal cord and brain

Seizure disorders, such as epilepsy

Cancer, such as brain tumors

Infections, such as meningitis[11]

Cancer is the uncontrolled growth of abnormal cells in the body. Cancerous cells are also called malignant cells.

Causes

Cells are the building blocks of living things. Cancer grows out of normal cells in the body. Normal cells multiply when the body needs them, and die when the body doesn't need them. Cancer appears to occur when the growth of cells in the body is out of control and cells divide too quickly. It can also occur when cells "forget" how to die.

There are many different kinds of cancers. Cancer can develop in almost any organ or tissue, such as the lung, colon, breast, skin, bones, or nerve tissue.

There are many causes of cancers, including:
  Benzene and other chemicals
  Certain poisonous mushrooms and a type of poison that can
    grow on peanut plants (aflatoxins)
  Certain viruses
  Radiation
  Sunlight
  Tobacco
  However, the cause of many cancers remains unknown.
  The most common cause of cancer-related death is lung
    cancer.

The three most common cancers in men in the United States are:
  Prostate cancer
  Lung cancer
  Colon cancer

In women in the U.S., the three most common cancers are:
  Breast cancer
  Colon cancer
  Lung cancer

Some cancers are more common in certain parts of the world. For
example, in Japan, there are many cases of gastric cancer, but in
the U.S. this type of cancer is pretty rare. Differences in diet may
play a role.

Some other types of cancers include:
  Brain cancer
  Cervical cancer
  Hodgkin's lymphoma
  Kidney cancer
  Leukemia
  Liver cancer

Non-Hodgkin's lymphoma
Ovarian cancer
Skin cancer
Testicular cancer
Thyroid cancer
Uterine cancer [12]

What is a metastasis or metastatic cancer?[13]

Metastasis and metastatic disease are terms used to describe cancer cells/tumours that have migrated to a new area of the body.

Most cancers start in one part of the body that is identified as the primary site. The type of cancer cells produced in this primary site can then migrate elsewhere. For example, breast cancer cells can migrate to the brain and grow into new "breast cancer" tumours in the brain. So, if the tumours in the brain are found before those in the breast, the primary site can be traced back to the breast. Finding the primary site helps doctors to identify the specific cancer, how long the disease has been present and what treatments are the best to use for the particular cancer.

Each cancer has a path that its metastasis (migrating cells) usually follows. It is called a "metastatic pathway". As the disease progresses, the cancer may show up in these predicted places and produce symptoms caused by the cancer affecting the new area.

Some common metastatic pathways:

Bladder: Local extension into pelvis, abdomen, also lung and bone

Brain: Brain tumours usually are the result of metastasis from some other primary site. Primary brain tumours such as glioblastoma and astrocytoma, do not usually spread elsewhere

Bone: Primary bone cancer is very rare. Tumours are usually the result of metastasis from some other primary site

Breast: Lymph nodes under the arm & chest walls, lungs, liver, bones & brain

Cervix/Uterus: Local extensions into the abdomen and pelvis

Esophagus: Chest, heart and lungs

Kidney: Bone, brain and lung

Liver: Tends to be a primary site that doesn't spread elsewhere

Lung: Brain, liver, bone, other lung

Ovary: Abdomen, pelvis

Pancreas: Stomach

Prostate: Bone, within the pelvis, brain and lung

Skin: Brain

Testes: Pelvis, abdomen, lung, liver, brain

At times when working with a client we may determine that they are not quite their normal happy selves, and when we enquire the reason, it is due to them being in pain.

While giving Reiki to a client can help relieve pain we also need to be aware of the different types of pain, and have knowledge of the current rating scales.

Pain can have negative effects on your body. Pain can affect your mental wellbeing, sleep patterns, your relationships, your ability to work, your posture and mobility, and it often affects your lifestyle choices. Pain may have caused you to avoid exercise, either out of fear of re-injury or because movement makes your pain worse. However, if you build up a regular exercise routine you can increase your strength, your stamina, and your flexibility and it could help you get back to some of the activities that you couldn't do because of your pain. Exercise programs have been helpful for people with back pain, fibromyalgia, neck pain, and other pain conditions. [14]

Acute pain is usually due to an injury, surgery or cancer and serves to protect us. When tissue is damaged, free nerve endings in your skin send signals to your brain via your spinal cord. Your brain then sends signals to your body to respond to pain, such as removing your burning finger from a hot stove.

Chronic pain is pain that persists over three months, beyond when an injury should have healed. Chronic pain can be intermittent (occurs in a pattern) or persistent (lasting more than 12 hours daily) and can be considered a disease itself. Usually the pain results from a known cause, such as surgery, or inflammation from arthritis. Sometimes the cause of this pain is abnormal processing of pain by the nervous system as in the case of fibromyalgia.

Pain signals to your brain may keep occurring long after the injury due to changes in the nervous system. This is called neuropathic pain. Many common diseases can result in changes in our nervous systems that cause pain. Shingles, diabetic neuropathies, and stroke are common examples.[15]

Should I try to ignore my pain? No! Today we know that pain should be treated instead of ignored. Good pain management can allow your body to heal and allow you to return to your normal activities, resulting in better quality of life.

Who can I turn to? Many people may be involved in helping you manage persistent pain. Some nurses specialize in pain management, as do physicians, physiotherapists, occupational therapists, and psychologists. Physiotherapy, psychological counseling, pain courses, meditation, and support groups may all play a role in helping to manage your pain. You also have the option of being referred by your family doctor to a pain specialist if your pain persists.

Treating pain requires a partnership between you and your healthcare professionals. Here are some tips for this partnership:

Keep a pain diary, recording the amount of pain, time which

pain was experienced, what you did to help the pain, and its effect. It is helpful to include the medications that you have taken and your activities. It can be useful in helping you to talk to your doctor about your pain. See the attached sample pain diary at the end of this booklet.

Describe your pain using words like throbbing, stabbing, burning, aching, tingling, dull, pressing, etc.

Rate your pain on a scale of 0-10, with 0 as no pain and 10 being the worst pain you can imagine.

List what you have tried already, what helps, what makes it worse.

Remember that you are the expert on your own body. You have the right to be listened to about your pain.

Bring a family member or friend along to medical visits to make sure you don't miss important information.

Continue to use medications as prescribed and discuss any concerns or side effects with your healthcare team.

Remember that you have the right to refuse a treatment option for your pain. You also have the right to have your pain reassessed regularly and your treatment adjusted if your pain has not been eased.[16]

The following is a description of the various pain scales that are used when rating cancer and non-cancer pain.

Pain assessment tools

Assessment is best performed using reliable and valid pain assessment scales and tools. Here are examples of some of the more commonly used scales and tools for both acute and chronic pain.

Standard pain assessment tools: Unidimensional tools

Some of the earliest pain assessment tools are one-dimensional pain scales, which were designed to measure pain intensity alone. Examples of this type of scale include the Visual Analog Scale (VAS), the Simple Descriptive Pain Intensity Scale (VDS), and the standard 0 to 10 Numeric Pain Intensity Scale (NPI).

A systematic review of 164 journal articles on pain indicates that single item ratings of pain intensity are valid and reliable measures of pain intensity (Jensen 2003).

Visual Analog Scale

The Visual Analog Scale (VAS) is a 100-millimeter line with "no pain" on one end and "pain as bad as it can be" at the other end. This scale is a very simple form of assessment. Patients are expected to mark on the line the amount of pain they are experiencing.

Patients with visual impairment find this scale difficult to use, and some elderly patients have difficulty marking on the line (Herr 1993, AHCPR 1994, D'Arcy 2003).

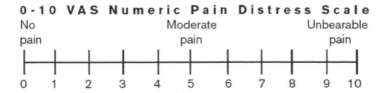

0 - 10 V A S N u m e r i c P a i n D i s t r e s s S c a l e

No pain	Moderate pain	Unbearable pain
0 1 2 3 4	5 6 7	8 9 10

Verbal Descriptor Scale

The Verbal Descriptor Scale (VDS) uses words such as "no pain," "moderate pain," or "worst possible pain" to help patients describe pain intensity. To use this scale, patients must be able to understand the use of the words and their meanings.

Feldt, Ryden, and Miles (1998) found a 73% completion rate

using this scale with a group of cognitively impaired patients. Additionally, some adults prefer using words to describe pain rather than numbers (Herr 1993, D'Arcy 2003).

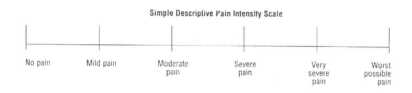

Simple Descriptive Pain Intensity Scale

| No pain | Mild pain | Moderate pain | Severe pain | Very severe pain | Worst possible pain |

Numeric Pain Intensity Scale

The most commonly used one-dimensional pain scale is the Numeric Pain Intensity Scale (NPI), also called the Numeric Rating Scale (NRS). This scale is made up of a horizontal line with the beginning point marked 0, or "no pain," and the opposite end marked 10, or "worst possible pain." Patients are asked to rate their pain from 0 to 10, choosing the number that best represents the intensity of the pain they are experiencing. Generally the pain in the 1–3 range is considered mild pain, 4–6 indicates moderate pain, and 7–10 is the highest level, or severe level, of pain.

This scale is useful for assessing efficacy of pain interventions. For example, by asking the patient for a numeric rating prior to pain medication and then asking the pain rating after half an hour or one hour, healthcare providers can measure the efficacy of the medication. A decrease of three points on the NPI is considered to be significant (Gordon et al, 2004)

There is no right or wrong number for patients to report. The nurse should ask the patient to rate the pain, and he or she should believe the number the patient reports.

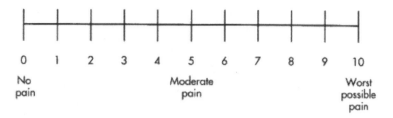

Using standard pain assessment scales

For acute pain, standard pain assessment scales work fairly well. But for patients with chronic pain who live with daily pain, numeric scales are more difficult to use. A better way for nurses to gauge improvement is to ask patients with chronic pain what level they experience on a daily basis. For these patients, success with pain management may need to be measured by the increase in a patient's functionality, rather than by the decrease in pain intensity (Pasero & McCaffery 2004).

Visual pain assessment tools and combined pain assessment scales

Thermometer scale

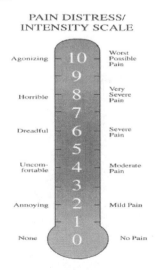

Some patients rate pain more easily when given a picture of the pain scale. The combined scale uses color—blue for less pain and red for more pain—and arranges the numbers in ascending order. For patients who have difficulty with numeric ratings, the verbal descriptors along the thermometer may help patients determine where the pain they are experiencing should be rated (D'Arcy 2003).[17]

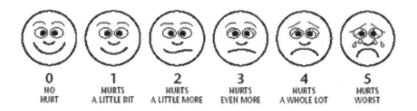

0	**1**	**2**	**3**	**4**	**5**
NO HURT	HURTS A LITTLE BIT	HURTS A LITTLE MORE	HURTS EVEN MORE	HURTS A WHOLE LOT	HURTS WORST

This scale uses faces to indicate intensity of pain.[18]

Note: with face number five you hurt as much as you can imagine, although you don't have to be crying to feel this bad.

When working with children or cognitively impaired adults and seniors we can use this scale.

Healing Crisis – Detox Reaction

"All cure starts from within out and from the head down and in reverse order as the symptoms have appeared".

(Hering's Law of Cure)

As previously mentioned Reiki appears to be generally safe, and no serious side effects have been reported. It has been my personal experience that 99.97% of my clients do not have a healing crisis/detox reaction. As an ethical Reiki practitioner it is important that we inform our client and their caregivers of this likelihood no matter how small. Some people would argue that the client might report a healing crisis because we have planted the thought in their mind that such a thing can happen. Our thoughts create our reality. Yes, this is a possibility however it does not matter. The practitioner needs to make the client and caregivers aware that symptoms of the ailment or condition being treated may get worse before getting better.

"Serious side effects from responsible hands-on energy inter-ventions are, in fact, rarely if ever seen, with the most frequently reported difficulties involving too much energy being moved too quickly for a physically unstable person to readily accommodate."[19]

A stagnation of energy can be akin to an energy block. This block in the client's body needs to be removed like when a drain gets clogged. The method that the practitioner uses is less drastic than a plumber's snake or Drano ©, but the effects are the same. During the reiki session some clients feel heat coming from the practitioner's hands, or they could experience cold, a pulse or even temporary pain. Reassure your client that these sensations are normal, and they will pass quickly. After the session the client may still be adjusting to this change in energy flow.

The healing crisis is nature's way of communicating with the individual that something is out of balance. It is the body itself that has the make-up and the materials that produce a crisis. It requires energy to have a crisis; it takes activity of blood cells and power of tissue structure. It takes a reserve to go through a healing crisis, and the body will not produce it, unless it is able to go through with it. We cannot put a new foundation in the body without first cleansing the body, sometimes the process is not always comfortable. It then provokes, say a cold, or some other mucous discharge to flush out the obstruction, calling in an army of macrophage and other immune defenders to help dispose of the stuff.

During a healing crisis, a great deal of toxins may be pulled out of body tissues and put back into the circulation in order to be eliminated. During this process, some uncomfortable symptoms may occur, such as:

general fatigue

pains and aches, such as headaches, low back pain, joint pain, etc.

skin discharges, unusual sweating and body odours

frequent urination, diarrhea or constipation

fever, or feeling of coldness

temporary cessation of menstruation, or decrease in sexual desire mental irritability, restless dreams, etc.

If a healing crisis occurs it may last from a few hours to a few days; only in extremely rare cases will it last a few weeks. The healthier our general condition, the fewer symptoms there will be. The more the body has to clean up, the stronger and / or the longer will be the discharge reactions. Support your body and this cleansing process by drinking quality water, eating more alkaline foods and staying away from white flour, white sugar and overly processed foods.

During the healing process, the body brings back old diseases in reverse order, especially if these diseases have been suppressed through medication. It is like a movie seen backwards. However, the eliminative processes may bring back old troubles in such a way that it inspires one to live an entirely different life, so that we are finished with that old way of living.

A better example might be a person with plantar fascitis. The person's feet hurt and they go to their family doctor. He recommends the person be fitted with orthotics. Once the orthotics are inserted into the person's shoes and they start walking, they notice that the feet still hurt. Until the muscles, tendons (etc.) get accustomed to you wearing the orthotics this sensation is not unusual.

Depending on the nature of the Reiki session a client may be asked to return for follow-up sessions. The general rule of thumb is four to six. Note this is not a hard and fast rule, take into consideration the needs of your client, and the condition as it may take less or more.

If an acute condition, longer sessions within a short time span are more beneficial than one session each week for a number of weeks.

A protocol for a client's chronic condition could be every day or a couple of times a week. Once again depending on the improvement, the frequency of Reiki sessions would change to once a week, then every two weeks and so on. Eventually the client will recover and no longer needs you.

Maintaining the protocol with your practitioner is important as each session builds upon the previous one resulting in a clearing of this stagnated energy.

When is a good time to stop giving Reiki, you may be wondering? The client or the caregivers have two options.

The client if well established on the road to recovery, the practitioner may suggest they take a Beginners Reiki course so they will be able to self-treat every day. In the case of the caregivers, if they are interested they can also take the Beginners Reiki course, and then they can share the gift of Reiki with their loved one and practice self care.

Receiving Reiki every day whether by doing self-treatments or being treated by a practitioner will not overwhelm the body, nor make it dependent on the practitioner like an addiction. Reiki helps to restore the body to homeostasis – a balanced condition.

Can We Be Friends And Professional?

Interesting question with no easy answer, there is a lot of grey.

How do you know when you have crossed a boundary in your Therapeutic Relationship?

Building relationships with clients is no different than forming friendships with strangers, which in a sense our clients are. Certain amounts of information are shared between the professional caregiver and the client and the family if in a hospice or palliative care setting in order to build that trust factor.

Depending on the nature of your relationship with your client and their family your close emotional attachment could trigger your own emotional (wounds) issues, impair your judgment as to what is best for the client, they become dependent on you and phone at inappropriate times.

If you discover that as the practitioner you have crossed that boundary and suddenly withdraw your services the client and the family may feel hurt and abandoned. This is why it is a good idea to set clear boundaries during your first visit.

In the event that something does happen, who do you talk to for moral guidance?

In a personal practice that may be difficult but being part of an interdisciplinary team talk to your direct supervisor.

But what happens and how do you dis-engage from these warm lovely people once the client dies?

Do you go to the funeral?

Will you still pet sit their dog?

What about the exchanging of Birthday and Christmas cards?

Should you 'friend' them on the social media site of Facebook?

(Remember Standard 7 part s – refuse any gift, favour or hospitality from clients…) While a gift card from the liquor store is inappropriate for you to accept, what about a box of chocolates? Yes, it is one of those shades of grey. Practice and caution make it easier to decide the right course of action.

As professionals we must gently break away and let these families get on with their lives. That doesn't mean that we don't care about them or wonder how they are doing. Not to appear cold or heartless, however, our role was to assist that client and the family, once this role is complete – no matter how hard – we must move on.

If needed schedule an appointment with a bereavement councillor and ask for debriefing assistance. Be gentle with yourself and book some Reiki time for you.

Chapter Review:

A lot of ground has been covered in this chapter with regards to sharing what Reiki is and how to compassionately care for a client. As you work with more clients and caregivers your communication: verbal and listening, and sensitivity skills will develop.

Be mindful of your scope of practice; ask for clarification when necessary and most of all enjoy the relationship you will cultivate with your client and their caregivers.

It may take some practice to get used to explaining the nature or possibility of a healing crisis/detox reaction. How comfortable are you in explaining this?

How will you distance yourself from the family once the client dies?

Chapter 7

Conclusion

The world of Complementary and Alternative Medicine (CAM) is changing and for that matter so is Modern Medicine. Our patients and/or clients are striving to make sense of their lives in this increasingly complex world and discover that it is not always easy to find balance on this tightrope of life.

Through the various chapters we have tried to understand the past, the present and hopefully create a positive future for CAM.

We know that energy is all around us; from that brilliant yellow orb in the sky we call our Sun to the small packets of energy (mitochondria, DNA, enzymes and chemical messengers) that assist our bodies in functioning as precisely as they do.

We have explored the concept of the body-mind from ancient days to modern times. It appears that the fragmentation of the self into those two aspects 'body' and 'mind' has lead to a broken telephone effect and the current state of affairs in health care. While our internal chemical/hormonal messengers have access to the whole body, our understanding of how our thoughts, feelings, and emotions interact with the physical body have been downplayed or even ignored.

When we look at the medical systems of other cultures, specifically Ayurvedic and Traditional Chinese, they look at the whole person to see what is out of balance and what steps need to be taken to restore that balance. Having this broader perspective combined with modern diagnostic tools can help validate what the ancients have known or what some might call anecdotal evidence.

Our colleagues in Modern Medicine are asked to uphold and maintain the highest quality standards in order to provide consistent quality care to their patients. We in the Complementary and Alternative Medicine fields also recognize that quality, consistent care is important. However, when an existing standard is trying to measure or quantify a substance or object that hasn't been identified by science the task is made more difficult.

What experiments can we devise to detect acupuncture meridians? We know what sound vibrations can do but what about subtle vibrations? What do they do? Exploring these and related topics hopefully will lead to acceptance and less derision regarding CAM therapies.

The onus is on all Complementary and Alternative practitioners to become familiar with and educated in the ways of confidentiality, cultural competence, ethics, standards and professionalism. Our clients are our partners in this medical paradigm shift and we need to be ready.

Thank you for sharing this journey, and radiant abundant health to everyone.

Appendix 1

Examples of pathogenic microbes and infectious diseases recognized since 1973

1973 Rotavirus Virus Major cause of infantile diarrhea worldwide

1975 Parvovirus Bl9 Virus Aplasticcrisisinchronichemolyticanemia

1976 Cryptosporidium parvum Parasite Acute and chronic diarrhea

1977 Ebola Virus Virus Ebola hemorrhagic fever

1977 Legionella pneumophila Bacteria Legionnaires' disease

1977 Hantaanvirus Virus Hemorragic fever with renal syndrome (HRFS)

1977 Campylobacter jejuni Bacteria Enteric pathogens distributed globally

1980 Human T-lymphotropic Virus T-cell lymphoma-leukemia virus I (HTLV-l)

1981 Toxic producing strains of Staphylococcus aureus Bacteria Toxic shock syndrome (tampon use)

1982 Escherichia coli 0157:H7 Bacteria Hemorrhagic colitis; hemolytic uremic syndrome

1982 HTLV-II Virus Hairy cell leukemia

1982 Borrelia burgdorferi Bacteria Lyme disease

1983 Human immunodeficiency virus (HIV) Virus Acquiredimmunodeficiency syndrome (AIDS)

1983 Helicobacter pylori Bacteria Peptic ulcer disease

1985 Enterocytozoon bieneusi Parasite Persistent diarrhea

1986 Cyclospora cayatanensis Parasite Persistent diarrhea

1988 Human herpesvirus-6 (HHV-6) Virus Roseola subitum

1988 Hepatitis E Virus Enterically transmitted non-A, non-B hepatitis

1989   Ehrlichia chafeensis Bacteria Human ehrlichiosis

1989   Hepatitis C Virus Parenterally transmitted non-A, non-B, liver infection

1991   Guanarito virus Virus Venezuelan hemorrhagic fever

1991   Encephalitozzon hellem Parasite Conjuncavitis, disseminated disease

1991   New species of Babesia Parasite Atypical babesiosis

1992   Vibrio cholerae 0139 Bacteria New strain associated with epidemic cholera

1992   Bartonella henselae Bacteria Cat-saatch disease;bacillaryangiomatosis

1993   Sin nombre virus Virus Adult respiratory distress syndrome

1993   Encephalitozoon cuniculi Parasite Disseminated disease

1994   Sabia virus Virus Brazilian hemolrhagic fever

1995   HHV-8 Virus Associated with Kaposi sarcoma in AIDS patients[1]

1 http://www.fas.org/promed/about/table2.html

Appendix 2

190   March 2000

Family Medicine

How to Write a Case Report

Laine H. McCarthy, MLIS; Kathryn E.H. Reilly, MD, MPH

Background: *Since before Hippocrates, case reports have provided a rich resource for teaching and research in medicine. Case reports are published by many prominent journals—more than 140,000 case reports are indexed in MEDLINE from 1996 to present—and a number of narrative guidelines for the preparation of case reports have appeared in the medical literature. To facilitate the preparation of case reports, we reviewed the existing guidelines and a random sampling of published case reports and created a fill-in-the-blanks worksheet for physicians to use to capture unique scientific observations. Although originally developed to assist family practice residents to write case reports, the case report worksheet can be used by physicians in any practice setting and any discipline to collect and report interesting, unusual, or newsworthy cases.*

(Fam Med 2000;32(3):190-5.)

[A] striking anecdote was the case of Phineas Gage, the man who had a 4-ft iron bar blown through his frontal lobes and whose immortal remains are now in the Harvard Museum . . . . Had it been realized that one could interfere with large masses of the cerebral hemispheres without killing the patient, and that great damage to the frontal lobes need cause no obvious intellectual defect, neurosurgery might have been conceived 40 years earlier.[1]

Since before Hippocrates, case reports have made a valuable contribution to the advancement of medical science.[1-9] A search of the MEDLINE database from 1996 to the present using the Medical Subject Heading (MeSH) term *case report* retrieved more than 140,000 citations. Several prominent medical journals have demonstrated an interest in increasing the number and quality of published case reports.[2-5,10-12]

Case reports are "scientific observations . . . that are carefully documented so that they may be a valuable education and research resource."[6] Sir William Osler, himself the author of many such scientific observations, encouraged other physicians to "Always note and record the unusual . . . . When you have made and recorded the unusual or original observation . . . publish it."[6] A case report, published in the *American Journal of*

Dermatopathology in 1981, was one of the first published accounts of what is now called AIDS.[13]

To help practitioners write case reports, we developed an outline-style worksheet. We began by searching the MEDLINE database from 1966 to the present using the MeSH terms *case report* and *publishing* to extract citations about writing case reports.[1-12,14-17] We also combined the term *case report* with keywords for various disciplines (eg, obstetrics and gynecology, pediatrics, neurology and neurosurgery, dermatology, general internal medicine, family medicine)[18-31] and selected a random sampling of published case reports. We studied these articles to determine the content and format that comprises published case reports.

The Content
What Kinds of Cases Should Be Reported
Much has been written about what type of case is worthy of reporting and publishing. Nathan[1] makes a strong case for reporting cases that "appeal to the emotions." He also points out that although an observation may be uncommon, unless it is reported, the frequency of its occurrence cannot be tabulated. Throughout history, reports of unusual cases have led to significant research and resulted in important clinical advances.[1,6,7,12,13] What guidelines, then, should a potential author use for deciding whether "this" case is significant enough to warrant writing?

To answer this difficult question, we reviewed previous published guidelines and examined the content of published case reports. Most case reports concern

From the Department of Family and Preventive Medicine, University of Oklahoma Health Sciences Center.

Vol. 32, No. 3 191

specialty and subspecialty topics that describe uncommon or unique clinical encounters, in keeping with the history of published case reports.[18,20,22,24,25,28,30,31] (Only 184 out of more than 140,000 case reports in the MEDLINE database from 1996 to the present are indexed under primary care.) Other cases, although reporting unusual outcomes or events, went on to describe lessons learned from patient interactions and interventions.[21,23,26,27,29,32-35] Clearly, there is room for both types of reports in the medical literature.

Our own review of published cases and existing guidelines suggest that case reports should describe a unique presentation, and its uniqueness should not simply be a variation from a previously reported case. For example, a new or unusual location for a previously recognized disease does not constitute a unique event unless it is accompanied by previously undocumented symptoms or unless it required a particularly lengthy and costly diagnostic process.[2,10,14]

Examples of observations that meet the uniqueness criteria are cases with characteristics such as those shown in Table 1.

Most existing guidelines were published in the specialty and subspecialty literature.[6,9,16] Two exceptions are a 1968 article in the *Journal of the American Medical Association*[15] by Roland, who represented the Scientific Publications Division of the American Medical Association, and Squires' 1989 article that appeared in the *Canadian Medical Association Journal*.[11] Both of these articles state that the purpose of case reporting is to describe the unique, newsworthy, or unusual. Since much of family practice is caring for common problems, and it is the unusual or unique presentation that forms the basis for a case report, it would seem appropriate for the editorial boards of the various family practice journals to define the criteria for accepting case reports and describe those criteria in their instructions to authors.

The Format

Components of a Case Report

Most previously published material about how to prepare case reports identified three major components: introduction, case presentation, and discussion.[11,14,15] Most also suggested that a brief, highly focused literature review be included, usually as part of the introduction. A detailed guideline for preparing a case report by DeBakey and DeBakey[16] expanded this format to five sections: introduction, description of the case, discussion, literature review, and summary/conclusions.

None of the previously published guidelines for case reports suggested the inclusion of an abstract, and few journals include abstracts in the case reports they publish. We advocate for the inclusion of an abstract (perhaps in lieu of the introduction) so that more information about the case can be retrieved from electronic databases such as MEDLINE. Since about 1970, the

Table 1

Characteristics of Cases Suitable
for Publication in a Case Report

- Cases that contribute to a change in the course of medical science[13]

- Cases that illustrate a new principle or support or refute a current theory and thus may stimulate research[16]

- Cases that present a therapeutic or diagnostic observation that elucidates a previously misunderstood clinical condition or response

- Cases that demonstrate an adverse response to drug therapies or presumed cause-and-effect presentations that have not been detected or reported[8,16]

- An unusual combination of conditions, cascading events,[33] or presenting complaints that confused the decision-making process or created treatment dilemmas.[26] The first reported cases of toxic shock syndrome involved a strange melange of presenting signs and symptoms that established the need for detailed clinical research.[8] A new observation of the impact of one disease process or condition on another, or of a treatment regime for one condition that results in an unexpected outcome of a different condition, are legitimate subjects for case reporting.[36]

- Reports that describe the personal influence a particular event had on the patient, the physician, or both. A case that causes a physician to reevaluate how he or she cared for patients[37] or a case that suggests opportunities for patient education are examples.[31]

MEDLINE record has included abstracts with all indexed articles that have an author-written abstract attached. Squires noted that for a case report to be worth writing and publishing, physicians must be able to "anticipate its interest and relevance to them and their practice."[11] Without an abstract available in an electronically searchable database, the likelihood that physicians will be able to anticipate the relevance of a particular case is diminished.

Taking all of the suggestions from previous published guidelines together with the structural components of several recently published reports and our own observations, we recommend that these five sections be included in a case report: 1) abstract/introduction, 2) case history/description, 3) literature review, 4) discussion, 5) conclusions/recommendations.

Although previously published guidelines have been thorough, they have mostly been narrative. Only one guideline offered a graphic representation of a case report—that guideline was prepared from the perspective of the reviewer, which would be an excellent resource for revising and editing a case paper once the first draft has been written but does not present enough detail to serve as a worksheet.[11] Using the five basic sections as a framework, we built a detailed outline or template that can be filled in by physicians interested in writing and publishing a case report. We call this template the case report worksheet (Figure 1). The following subsections describe the content of each field

192   March 2000   *Family Medicine*

Figure 1

Case Report Worksheet (Content of a Case Report)

Author (s) _____

Title _____

1) Abstract
   Clinical question/problem _____
   Analysis of literature review _____
   Summary _____

2) Case history/report
   A. Description of patient _____
   B. History of presenting condition _____
   C. Physical exam _____
   D. Relevant lab/X ray/other tests _____
   E. Initial diagnosis and treatment _____
   F. Expected outcome _____
   G. Actual outcome _____

3) Literature search
   A. MEDLINE/other database _____
   B. Search terms _____
   C. Results of search (# relevant, citations, what you learned) _____

4) Discussion (significance, why you're writing this)
   A. Relevant literature _____
   B. Hypothesis _____
   C. Diagnostic process/course of illness _____
      i.   Table of diagnostic process _____
      ii. Figures, photographs, imaging _____
   D. Outcomes _____
      i.   Drug-drug interactions _____
      ii. Drug-condition interactions _____
      iii. Other conflicting outcomes/observations _____

5) Conclusions/recommendations (lesson learned) _____
   _____
   _____
   _____
   _____

References _____
   _____
   _____

of the template and provide examples to facilitate preparation of a case report using the worksheet.

1) Abstract

Along with the title, abstracts are an important component of the electronic bibliographic record of each article in databases such as MEDLINE. Abstracts allow readers to quickly scan the content of an article to determine whether it is sufficiently relevant to merit further reading. Without abstracts, many articles that may be pertinent to a clinical situation may be overlooked.

In lieu of or in addition to an introduction, we suggest adding a brief abstract that contains the clinical question or problem, an analysis of the literature review, and a brief statement summarizing why this case is unusual and noteworthy. Here is an example of an abstract of less than 100 words:

A 10 year-old-boy presented with a 4-year history of recurrent perioral rash. A MEDLINE search to answer the question, "What could cause intractable perioral rash in a 10-year-old-boy?" yielded several case reports describing unusual perioral rashes caused by the ingredients found in toothpaste. Given the history and unique pattern of the rash, the diagnosis of contact dermatitis caused by allergy to toothpaste was made. Minimal lifestyle changes resulted in resolution of the rash. Toothpaste allergy may be more common than currently thought, because of the difficulty of arriving at the diagnosis.

2) Case History/Report

The second section is the case history or case report, which is typically drawn from chart notes and is a central part of published case reports. It should begin with an introduction to the patient(s) and should provide a history of the current situation. Details about the physical exam and any test results that provide insights into the current case should be included, but authors should refrain from providing all test results and should be careful not to include "red herrings" unless they are likely to cause problems for other physicians.[14] Include normal laboratory values for less commonly ordered laboratory tests.[11,14,16] The goal is to include only the essential information to emphasize the striking features of the case.[14] The initial diagnosis and treatment and follow-up plan should be included in this section.[28] Tables,[26] flow charts,[28] photographs,[20,25,28,31] radiographs,[18,21] and figures,[30,31] can be included to elucidate the case.

3) Literature Review

The methods section for case reports is the formal, structured literature search, similar to that described for systematic reviews.[36] A well-built clinical question should be formulated,[39,40] followed by a description of the index terms or MeSH headings used for the searches,

so others can reproduce the search. For example, MeSH terms to answer the clinical question, "In a 10-year-old boy, what are the possible causes of intractable perioral rash?" might be "dermatitis, perioral" or "facial dermatoses." The literature review itself should be brief and concise, designed to assure the uniqueness of the case and to provide a backdrop for and the position of the new information in the biomedical literature.

Many editors and authors of guidelines caution against structuring or titling manuscripts as "A Case Report and Review of the Literature."[10,11] Case reports and literature reviews are two distinctly different article forms serving different information needs. Although a concise overview of the pertinent literature is necessary in a case report, a full-scale literature review is not relevant to the clinical question and the purpose of the case report, and it defies the critical need for case reports to be brief. All citations should be included at the end of the manuscript following the format required for the journal. (See "Barriers" below for a more complete discussion of the publication process.)

4) Discussion

The discussion section is the most important section of a case report. This is where the authors state the significance of the information. What about this patient was striking or unusual? Why is writing this up important? What will your colleagues learn? Note that not all subsets of the discussion section on the worksheet (Figure 1) will apply to all cases being reported. Choose the areas that best help elucidate your case, paying attention to the two watchwords of case reporting: brevity and clarity.[11,14] Most published case reports are less than three journal pages in length, and the vast majority are one page or less.

The discussion section should discuss the relevant literature in the context of the current case, describing why the case being reported is a new and noteworthy or unique observation. A hypothesis about the new condition might be generated to present the new information in relation to existing information.[9] The manner in which the data (scientific observations) were collected and assembled (eg, a chronology of events from the perspective of the physician or the patient) should be described as part of the diagnostic/revelation process. A short decision tree or algorithm might also be useful. Graphics can serve to replace words in these brief publications. A discussion of the outcomes of the case should be included. This section should justify the publication of the case report.

5) Summary/Conclusions/Recommendations Section

Finally, the paper should include a brief summary, conclusion, or recommendations section—the take-home message. Lessons the physician learned from caring for this patient—family, social or quality-of-life lessons, physician-patient communication barriers, or compliance issues[37]—should be described in this section. Ask questions like, "What would I do differently next time now that I've had this experience?" or "What recommendations can I offer to other clinicians?" Recommendations for research should also be included. This section should likewise be brief, generally only one or two paragraphs.

Overcoming Barriers to Writing Case Reports

Practitioners interested in writing case reports or other manuscripts for publication face a number of barriers. The greatest barrier is time. The case report worksheet can streamline the process of writing a case report by directing the clinician's data collection (those scientific observations that comprise a case report). Once completed, the notes and observations can be readily formatted into a manuscript for submission.

Another obstacle is that practitioners may be intimidated by the publication process. The guideline published by DeBakey and DeBakey provides a simple and thorough discussion of the publication process.[16] This guideline is especially useful for the novice author who would like a more in-depth discussion of the publication process than a more-experienced writer might need.

The case report worksheet has categories for all material appropriate for a brief case report (although not all information on the worksheet is appropriate for all topics) in a standard publication format. Instructions to authors for the journal should be consulted early in the writing process, so the manuscript can be prepared in the appropriate style. All journals print instructions for authors regularly,[41,42] and many journals now publish their instructions on-line (eg, www.stfm.org/instruct.html and www.abfp.org/journal.htm). The "Uniform Requirements for Manuscripts Submitted to Biomedical Journals" form the basis for most journal instructions and should be consulted to answer format and content questions not addressed by the journal's instructions.[43] The "Uniform Requirements" are also available on-line at the American Medical Association Web site (jama.ama-assn.org/info/auinst.html).

When the manuscript is received by the journal, it will go through a brief editorial review to determine potential suitability for the journal, followed, if appropriate, by a peer-review process, during which reviewers comment on the article's significance and its relevance to the journal's scope and readership. While many manuscripts are rejected, some are returned to the author with an invitation to revise and resubmit the manuscript for further consideration. The comments from reviewers help authors revise and edit manuscripts, which can then resubmitted for publication. A detailed letter to the editor describing how the reviewer's comments were addressed should accompany the revised manuscript.

Table 2

Partial Listing of Primary Care Journals
That Accept and Publish Case Reports

Academic Emergency Medicine

American Family Physician

Archives of Family Medicine

Archives of Internal Medicine

Journal of Family Practice

Journal of the American Board of Family Practice

Lancet

New England Journal of Medicine

A final obstacle is that physicians may not know which publications accept case reports. In Table 2, we have listed several primary care journals that publish case reports. *The New England Journal of Medicine* accepts case reports in the form of letters to the editor.[36] In addition, many local and state medical associations publish case reports,[44] as do specialty journals.[30,31] *Pediatrics* publishes many case reports as e-pages (electronic pages) on its Web site (www.pediatrics.org).[35]

Summary

The case report worksheet was designed to help guide the process of collecting observations of unusual cases in a scientific and structured manner and to overcome some of the barriers and anxieties physicians might encounter when preparing case reports. Adjusting the previously accepted structure of case reports (introduction/discussion/conclusion) to include an abstract and a brief literature review increases the usefulness and retrievability of case reports.

Case reports must be brief, present new or unique material, and follow a standard, structured approach to organizing and presenting clinical observations. Editors and editorial boards for primary care and family medicine journals should determine the specific criteria for accepting case reports (type of report, length, etc) and print those criteria in the instructions for authors for each journal. The case report worksheet provides a uniform approach to preparing case reports and can be used to collect and organize scientific observations into interesting and publishable case reports.

Acknowledgment: This work was presented at the 1999 Society of Teachers of Family Medicine Annual Spring Conference in Seattle.

Corresponding Author: Address correspondence to Ms McCarthy, University of Oklahoma Health Sciences Center, Department of Family and Preventive Medicine, 900 NE 10th Street, Oklahoma City, OK 73104. 405-271-2374. Fax: 405-271-2784. E-mail: laine-mccarthy@ouhsc.edu.

REFERENCES

1. Nathan PW. When is an anecdote? Lancet 1967;2:607.
2. Pascal RR. Case reports—desideratum or rubbish? Hum Pathol 1985;16:759.
3. Rightmaier WJ. Case report. Arch Otolaryngol Head Neck Surg 1993;119:926.
4. Friedell MT. The case report. Int Surg 1973;58:225.
5. Morgan PP. Why case reports? Can Med Assoc J 1985;133:353.
6. Coccia CT, Ausman JI. Is a case report an anecdote? In defense of personal observations in medicine. Surg Neurol 1987;28:111-3.
7. Treasure T. What is the place of the clinical case report in medical publishing? J R Soc Med 1995;88:279.
8. Morris BA. The importance of case reports. Can Med Assoc J 1989;141:875-6.
9. Simpson RJ Jr, Griggs TR. Case reports and medical progress. Perspect Biol Med 1985;28:402-6.
10. Soffer A. Case reports in the *Archives of Internal Medicine.* Arch Intern Med 1976;136:1090.
11. Squires BP. Case reports: what editors want from authors and peer reviewers. Can Med Assoc J 1989;141:379-80.
12. Riesenberg DE. Case reports in the medical literature. JAMA 1986;255:2067.
13. Gottlieb GJ, Rogoz A, Vogel JV, et al. A preliminary communication on extensively disseminated Kaposi's sarcoma in a young homosexual man. Am J Dermatopathol 1981;3:111-4.
14. Riley HD. Preparing a case report. South Med J 1975;68:79-80.
15. Roland CG. The case report. JAMA 1968;205:83-4.
16. DeBakey L, DeBakey S. The case report. I. Guidelines for preparation. Int J Cardiol 1983;4:357-64.
17. DeBakey L, DeBakey S. The case report. II. Style and form. Int J Cardiol 1983;6:247-54.
18. Arakawa K, Akita T, Nishizawa K, et al. Anticoagulant therapy during successful pregnancy and delivery in a Kawasaki disease patient with coronary aneurysm: a case report. Japanese Circulation Journal 1997;61:197-200.
19. Pasternak AV IV, Graziano FM. Neurosarcoidosis: case report and brief literature review. J Am Board Fam Pract 1999;12:406-8.
20. Bradway MW, Drezner AD. Popliteal aneurysm presenting as acute thrombosis and ischemia in a middle-aged man with a history of Kawasaki disease. J Vasc Surg 1997;26:884-7.
21. Embil JM, Kramer M, Kinnear S, Light RB. A blinding headache. Lancet 1997;350:182.
22. Hanzlick R, Nicohols L. The Autopsy Committee of the College of American Pathologists. Case of the month: mycobacterium tuberculosis. Arch Intern Med 1998;158:426.
23. Hart AL, Kamm MA, Palmer JG, Talbot IC. An extraordinary cause of megacolon. Lancet 1997;350:110.
24. Lee EY, Cibull ML, Hanzlick R. The Autopsy Committee of the College of American Pathologists. Case of the month: drug hypersensitivity reaction. Arch Intern Med 1997;157:2044.
25. Matfin G, Berger KW, Adelman HM. Milky ascites in a former whiskey runner. Hosp Pract 1997;Aug 15:39-40,43.
26. Melberg A, Mattsson P, Westerberg CE. Loss of control after a cup of coffee. Lancet 1997;350:1220.
27. Sarkisian EC, Boiko S, Hood AF. Acute localized bullous eruption in a boy. Arch Fam Med 1998;7:11-2.
28. Walker IS, Hogan DE. Bite to the left leg. Acad Emerg Med 1995;2:223, 231-7.
29. Welch KMA. A 27-year-old woman with migraine headaches. JAMA 1997;278:322-8.
30. Sauerbrei A, Müller D, Eichhorn U, Wutzler P. Detection of varicellazoster virus in congenital varicella syndrome: a case report. Obstet Gynecol 1996;88:687-9.
31. Ruvalcaba RHA, Kletter GB. Abdominal lipohypertrophy caused by injections of growth hormone: a case report. Pediatrics 1998;102:408-10.
32. Schneeweiss R. Morning rounds and the search for evidence-based answers to clinical questions. J Am Board Fam Pract 1997;10:298-300.
33. Lawler MK, Olay MP, Ramakrishnan K, Barton ED. Lions and tigers and bears, oh my! Fam Med 1998;30:329-31.
34. Reilly KEH, McCarthy LH. Toothpaste allergy presenting as intractable perioral rash in a 10-year-old boy. J Am Board Fam Pract 2000;13:73-5.
35. Huff GF, Bagwell SP, Bachman D. Airbag injuries in infants and children: a case report and review of the literature. Pediatrics 1998;102:2.
36. Velasco M, Morán A, Téllez MJ. Resolution of chronic hepatitis B after ritonavir treatment in an HIV-infected patient. N Engl J Med 1999;340:1765-6.
37. Mold JW, McCarthy LH. Pearls from geriatrics, or a long line at the bathroom. J Fam Pract 1995;41:22-3.
38. Cook DJ, Mulrow CD, Haynes RB. Systematic reviews: synthesis of best evidence for clinical decisions. Ann Intern Med 1997;126:376-80.
39. Richardson WS, Wilson MC, Nishikawa J, Hayward RSA. The well-built clinical question: a key to evidence-based decisions. ACP J Club 1995;123:A-12-A-13.
40. Counsell C. Formulating questions and locating primary studies for inclusion in systematic reviews. Ann Intern Med 1997;127:380-7.
41. *Family Medicine* instructions to authors. Fam Med 1999;31:509-12.
42. Information for authors. J Am Board Fam Pract 1999;12:101-3.
43. Uniform requirements for manuscripts submitted to biomedical journals. JAMA 1997;277:927-34.
44. Guo X, Dick L. Late onset angiotensin-converting, enzyme-induced angioedema: case report and review of the literature. J Okla State Med Assoc 1999;92:71-3.

Appendix 3

30 January 2000 Family Medicine
Residency Education *Vol. 32, No. 1 31*

Suggested Curriculum Guidelines on Complementary and Alternative Medicine: Recommendations of the Society of Teachers of Family Medicine Group on Alternative Medicine

Benjamin Kligler, MD, MPH; Andrea Gordon, MD; Marian Stuart, PhD;
Victor Sierpina, MD

Background and Objectives: The widespread use of alternative and complementary therapies by the public provides a new challenge to medical education. No standardized curriculum is available for medical educators in this field. Providing an adequate background on these therapies and reliable, useful information to our learners was a task addressed by the Society of Teachers of Family Medicine (STFM) Group on Alternative Medicine over the past 2 years. Methods: The group met at conferences and communicated via e-mail to develop a consensus of recommended knowledge, skills, and attitudes in complementary and alternative medicine for incorporation into the family practice residency training curriculum. Conclusion: This article suggests guidelines as developed by this STFM group to assist programs wishing to include formal training in complementary and alternative medicine in residency training.
(Fam Med 1999;31(10):30-3.)

In response to the growing public interest in complementary /alternative approaches to health care, [1-4] patients' requests and media coverage have sparked physicians' interest in the potential applications of alternative therapies. A 1995 survey conducted by the Society of Teachers of Family Medicine (STFM) Group on

Alternative Medicine found that more than 28% of family practice residencies were including formal teaching on this topic in their curricula, [5] and it is likely that the percentage has increased since the time of that survey. Until now however, no formal guidelines have been developed to define which elements of the enormous field of alternative medicine should be included in the education of a family physician. This absence of a defined curriculum in complementary and alternative medicine (CAM) is also evident at the medical school level.[6]

Over the past 2 years, the STFM Group on Alternative Medicine has developed a set of suggested CAM curriculum guidelines for family practice residencies. These suggested guidelines are meant to provide an overview of key elements to be covered in a curriculum, rather than establishing specific training requirements. Although we recommend that all family practice residencies begin to introduce teaching on alternative medicine at some level into their curricula, it is clear that the depth to which a given program will follow these guidelines will depend on the skills and interest of the faculty of that program, as well as on the demand for and interest in alternative medicine in a residency's patient population.

The guidelines indicate the knowledge, skills, and attitudes that graduating residents should acquire to be able to function as unbiased advocates and advisors to patients about CAM. To communicate effectively with patients about alternative therapies requires that our graduates have a reasonable knowledge base in this area. They must be aware of which elements of CAM practice are based on adequate research evidence and which remain unproven. A willingness to discuss alternative therapies with patients and to admit our lack of knowledge are also essential.[7]

Curriculum Guidelines in Complementary/Alternative Medicine

A. Attitudes

A curriculum in complementary/alternative medicine (CAM) should educate residents to:

1. Understand and respect cultural/ethnic influences on health beliefs and health care choices, to include patients desiring "traditional" cultural and ethnic approaches to therapy and healing.
2. Discuss patients' use of complementary therapies as a necessary part of finding a common ground when practicing patient-centered medicine.
3. Respect the potential of certain complementary therapies to be equally or perhaps more effective than conventional approaches for the treatment of certain conditions.
4. Demonstrate willingness to seek out and collaborate with practitioners of complementary therapies to ensure patients' access to quality CAM when appropriate for their medical care.
5. Understand that physicians' attitudes toward their own self-care, self-awareness, and personal growth play a critical role in promoting the process of change in patients' lives.
6. Understand the role that physicians' own core beliefs and cultural, ethnic, or religious background may play in their choice of recommendations regarding their treatments.

B. Knowledge Residents should acquire:

1. Prevalence and patterns of use of CAM
a. Regional variation, particularly patterns within one's own area/community
b. Ethnic and cultural issues and the role of the patient's social system in determining health beliefs and choices
c. Conditions for which patients most commonly seek out complementary approaches

2. Legal issues regarding referral, collaboration with unconventional practitioners, and appropriate documentation

3. Current status of insurance reimbursement for CAM therapies in their area

4. Applications of the principles of evidence-based medicine to the study of CAM

5. Training, licensing, and credentialing standards for practitioners of chiropractic, acupuncture, massage therapy, and naturopathy. These licensing issues are often state-specific.

6. Modalities: for each of the CAM therapies listed below, residents will be able to describe:

a. The basic theory/philosophy of the discipline and the ways in which that philosophy diverges from the philosophy underlying conventional medicine

b. The common clinical applications and indications for referral

c. The potential for adverse effects

d. The current research evidence for efficacy and cost-effectiveness, including an awareness of the methodological issues and difficulties raised in studying the modality

e. One reputable reference source for more in-depth information

i. Mind/body medicine, including Ericksonian hypnotherapy, biofeedback, meditation, use of imagery and visualization, use of ceremony and ritual

ii. Alternative systems/culturally-based healing traditions, including at minimum, traditional Chinese medicine, including acupuncture and herbology, homeopathy, and Ayurvedic medicine. Residents should also have a basic understanding of the systems of traditional medicine practiced by the patient population in their area (eg, Native American, Asian-American, Latin American, etc)

iii. Manual therapy, manipulation, and energetic systems, including massage, chiropractic, osteopathic manipulation, therapeutic touch, and movement therapies such as Qi Gong

iv. Diet, nutrition, and lifestyle therapies, including specific nutritional interventions for certain conditions and the use of dietary supplements

v. Herbal medicine, including the European/North American herbal tradition

C. Skills

Residents should develop the following abilities:

1. Ability to inquire into patients' use of complementary therapies in a nonthreatening, nonjudgmental manner.

2. Ability to gather relevant information (when available) regarding safety, efficacy, and cost of a complementary therapies intervention and to communicate this information clearly to the patient

3. Ability to assist the patient in how to use conventional and complementary therapies in concert for maximum benefit, ie, to integrate the use of conventional and unconventional options in clinical practice

4. Ability to use the available data to help patients choose between a variety of CAM options for a given condition

5. Ability to interact with practitioners of CAM in a collegial manner to facilitate quality patient care

6. Ability to evaluate the strengths, weaknesses, and appropriate applications of a range of research methodologies to the area of CAM

7. Depending on the skills of the available faculty, residents may choose to develop specific skills in one or more of the following areas for application in their clinical practice:

a. Herbal medicine: use Western herbs safely and appropriately for treatment of common conditions for which they have been demonstrated to be helpful (eg, Saw Palmetto for BPH14).

b. Nutritional medicine: use vitamin/mineral supplements

appropriately for conditions where they have proven benefit (eg, Vitamin E for prevention of heart disease).Use dietary manipulation for treatment of certain conditions such as irritable bowel syndrome.

c. Mind/body medicine: use guided imagery and/or progressive relaxation techniques for stress-related conditions. Perform a "basic spiritual assessment" and understand when and how to refer for spiritual counseling. Use Ericksonian hypnotherapy techniques for smoking cessation.

d. Manipulation: use basic muscle energy/soft tissue and/or acupressure techniques for low-back pain, shoulder pain, neck pain, and headache. Teach a set of basic Qi Gong exercises.

e. Homeopathy: use of 5–10 common remedies for acute care situations

f. Acupuncture: elective time might be used to pursue the study of medical acupuncture through one of the several available courses.

In devising the CAM guidelines, the group used the format for educational guidelines developed by the American Academy of Family Physicians. For the sake of consistency with others writing in this area, we also incorporated the National Institutes of Health/Office of Alternative Medicine classification system for describing the categories of complementary/alternative therapies. CAM can be seen as an extension of a multicultural perspective consonant with the philosophical basis of family medicine and, as such, could ultimately become an established part of the family practice residency curriculum.

Implementation

A number of family practice residencies around the country are already implementing curricula based in whole or in part on these guidelines. The extent to which they will be implemented in a given program will depend on a number of local factors, including the skills and interests of the faculty, availability of reputable CAM practitioners, the general attitude of local physicians and the public regarding CAM practitioners, and the relative priority assigned to this content area in a program's overall curriculum. Often, the development of curricula in this area is dependent on a single faculty member with an interest and commitment.[8]

It remains to be seen what teaching strategy will be the most effective way to incorporate the use of complementary therapies into family practice residency training.

Faculty in various programs are currently experimenting with both intensive block experience and longitudinal strategies. One challenge to incorporating this teaching into a longitudinal outpatient experience is that many family medicine faculties, although interested in CAM, lack knowledge and skills in CAM and may not be comfortable in teaching and precepting residents on this topic. For this reason, faculty development must be the first priority for a program seeking to implement a curriculum in CAM. General definitions, as well as philosophical issues, are as essential to this faculty development effort as is the acquisition of specific skills.[9]

Another challenge is the need for more research into the safety and efficacy of many alternative therapies.[10]

As in many areas of conventional therapy, the quality of research needed for evidence-based assessment of CAM is often lacking.[11-13] As new studies emerge, the curriculum will necessarily evolve to reflect the growing body of scientific evidence in this field.

We have tried to emphasize in the guidelines that we do not advocate an unrestrained acceptance of any CAM therapies. Rather, each faculty member should be prepared to make a critical assessment of alternative treatments in the context of a patient's life and health issues.

There is also a need to evaluate the success or failure of our curricular initiatives in producing family physicians who are comfortable in discussing alternative therapies with patients. Residency programs should take a rigorous approach to evaluating their teaching efforts in this area.

Summary

Public interest in and use of complementary and alternative therapies continue to grow. Given this interest, we feel that family physicians have a responsibility to their patients to develop a basic understanding of the principles and applications of CAM in primary care.

As the group developed these guidelines, it became clear that in many ways, the inquiry of the family physician into the use of complementary therapies is a natural extension of the philosophic basis of family medicine and an application of the biopsychosocial perspective in which our training is grounded. The recommended guidelines outlined above should serve as an aid to family practice residencies undertaking the challenge of integrating teaching on complementary and alternative therapies into their curricula.

Corresponding Author: Address correspondence to Dr Kligler, Beth Israel Department of Family Medicine, 16 East 16th Street, New York, NY 10003.

212-206-5232. Fax: 212-206-5251. E-mail: benklig@aol.com.

References

1. Astin JA. Why patients use alternative medicine: results of a national study. JAMA 1998;279:1548-53.

2. Eisenberg D, Kessler R. Unconventional medicine in the United States. Prevalence, costs, and patterns of use. N Engl J Med 1993;328:246-52.

3. Eisenberg D, Davis RB, Ettner SL, et al. Trends in alternative medicine use in the United States, 1990–1997. JAMA 1998;280:1569-75.

4. Landmark Healthcare. The Landmark report on public perceptions of alternative care. Sacramento, Calif: Landmark Healthcare, 1998.

5. Carlson M, Stuart M, Jonas W. Alternative medicine instruction in medical schools and family practice residency programs. Fam Med 1997;29:559-62.

6. Wetzel MS, Eisenberg DM, Kaptchuk TJ. Courses involving complementary and alternative medicine at US medical schools. JAMA 1998;280:784-7.

7. Eisenberg D. Advising patients who seek alternative medical therapies. Ann Intern Med 1977;127(1):61-9.

8. Durso C. Special report, complementary and alternative medicine. The New Physician 1998;Nov:12-23.

9. Working Group on Definitions and Descriptions of Complementary Medicine. Defining and describing complementary and alternative medicine. Altern Ther Health Med 1997;3(2):49-57.

10. Angell M, Kassirer JP. Alternative medicine—the risks of untested and unregulated remedies (editorial). N Engl J Med 1998;339(12):839-41.

11. Jonas WB. Evaluating unconventional medical practices. Journal of the National Institutes of Health Research 1993;5:64-7.

12. Dossey L. How should alternative therapies be evaluated? An examination of fundamentals. Altern Ther Health Med 1995;1(2):6-10,79-85.
13. Levin JS, Glass TA, Kushi LH, et al. Qualitative methods in research on complementary and alternative medicine—a methodological manifesto. Med Care 1997,35(11):1079-94.
14. Wilt TJ, Ishani A, Stark G, et al. Saw palmetto extracts for treatment of benign prostatic hyperplasia. JAMA 1998;280:1604-9.

http://www.stfm.org/fmhub/Fullpdf/Jan00/re1.pdf (as of July 09)

Appendix 4

Learning to Write Case Notes Using the SOAP Format

Susan Cameron and imani turtle-song

This article discusses how to use the SOAP (subjective, objective, assessment, and plan) note format to provide clear and concise documentation of the client's continuum of care. Not only does this format allow for thorough documentation, but it also assists the counselor in representing client concerns in a holistic framework, thus permitting practitioners, paraprofessionals, and case managers to better understand the concerns and needs of the client. Whereas counselors working in certain settings (e.g., public funded institutions) are likely to find various recommendations in the article easy to incorporate into their current practice, the authors believe the recommendations are relevant to a wide array of settings.

In every mental health treatment facility across the country, counselors are required to accurately document what has transpired during the therapeutic hour. Over the course of the past few years, the importance of documentation has gained more emphasis as third-party payers have changed the use of documentation "from something that *should* be done well to something that *must* be done well" (Kettenbach, 1995, p. iii). In this era of accountability, counselors are expected to be both systematic in providing client services (Norris, 1995) and able to produce clear and comprehensive documentation of those clinical services rendered (Scalise, 2000). However, in my experience (i.e., first author), both as director of a mental health clinic and as one who audits client records, few counselors are able to write clear or concise clinical case notes, and most complain of feeling frustrated when trying to distinguish what is and is not important enough to be incorporated in these notes. Well-written case notes provide accountability, corroborate the delivery of appropriate services, support clinical decisions (Mitchell, 1991; Scalise, 2000), and, like any other skill, require practice to master. This article discusses how to accurately document rendered services and how to support clinical treatment decisions.

When counselors begin their work with the client, they need to ask themselves, What are the mental health needs of this client and how can they best be met? To answer this question, the counselor needs an organized method of planning, giving, evaluating, and recording rendered client services. A viable method of record keeping is SOAP noting (Griffith & Ignatavicius, 1986; Kettenbach, 1995). SOAP is an acronym for subjective (S), objective (O), assessment (A), and plan (P), with each initial letter representing one of the sections of the client case notes.

SOAP notes are part of the problem-oriented medical records (POMR) approach most commonly used by physi-

cians and other health care professionals. Developed by Weed (1964), SOAP notes are intended to improve the quality and continuity of client services by enhancing communication among the health care professionals (Kettenbach, 1995) and by assisting them in better recalling the details of each client's case (Ryback, 1974; Weed, 1971). This model enables counselors to identify, prioritize, and track client problems so that they can be attended to in a timely and systematic manner. But more important, it provides an ongoing assessment of both the client's progress and the treatment interventions. Although there are alternative case note models, such as data, assessment, and plan (DAP), individual educational programs (IEP), functional outcomes reporting (FOR), and narrative notes, all are variations of the original SOAP note format (Kettenbach, 1995).

To understand the nature of SOAP notes, it is essential to comprehend where and how they are used within the POMR format. POMRs consist of four components: database, problem list, initial plans, and SOAP notes (Weed, 1964). In many mental health facilities, the components of the POMR are respectively referred to as clinical assessment, problem list, treatment plan, and progress notes (Shaw, 1997; Siegal & Fischer, 1981). The *first* component, the clinical assessment, contains information gathered during the intake interview(s). This generally includes the reason the client is seeking treatment; secondary complaints; the client's personal, family, and social histories; psychological test results, if any; and diagnosis and recommendations for treatment (Piazza & Baruth, 1990). According to the Joint Commission on Accreditation of Healthcare Organizations (JCAHO, 2000), with special populations, as in the case of a child, the clinical assessment contains a developmental history; for individuals who present with a history of substance abuse, a drug and alcohol evaluation is included.

From the clinical assessments, a problem list (*second* component) is generated, which includes an index of all the problems, active or inactive, derived from the client's history. Problems

Susan Cameron, *Santa Fe Indian Hospital, Santa Fe, New Mexico;* **imani turtle-song**, *PB & J Family Services, Albuquerque, New Mexico. Correspondence concerning this article should be addressed to imani turtle-song, PB & J Family Services, 1101 Lopez SW, Albuquerque, NM 87105 (e-mail: imanisong@aol.com).*

are defined as either major areas of concern for the client that are not within the usual parameters when compared with others from the client's same age group or as areas of client concern that can be changed through therapeutic intervention (JCAHO, 2000). As problems are identified, they are numbered, dated, and entered on the list, and this problem list is attached to the inside cover of the client's file, for easy reference. As the identified problems are resolved, they are dated and made "inactive."

The *third* component of the POMR is the treatment plan, which is a statement of the possible therapeutic strategies and interventions to be used in dealing with each noted problem. Treatment plans are stated as goals and objectives and are written in behavioral terms in order to track the client's therapeutic progress, or lack thereof (Kettenbach, 1995). The priority of each objective is expressed either as a long or a short-term goal and corresponds to the problems list. Long-term goals are the expected final results of counseling, whereas short-term goals are those that can be accomplished within the next session or within a very limited time frame.

The *fourth* component is the progress notes, which are generally written using the SOAP format and serve to bridge the gap between the onset of counseling services and the final session. Using the SOAP format, the counselor is able to clearly document and thus support, through the subjective and objective sections, his or her decision to modify existing treatment goals or to fine-tune the client's treatment plan. For example, if a client who has been in counseling for 4 months experiences the unexpected death of a loved one or is diagnosed with a potentially life threatening health problem, by recording this information in the progress notes the counselor provides justification/documentation for the sudden shift in therapeutic direction and is immediately able to address what is now the more pressing issue for the client.

The SOAP note format also provides a problem-solving structure for the counselor. Because SOAP notes require adequate documentation to verify treatment choices, they serve to organize the counselor's thinking about the client and to aid in the planning of quality client care. For example, if the plan is to refer the client to a domestic violence group for perpetrators, the subjective and objective sections of the SOAP notes would chronicle the client's history of physical aggression and violent behaviors, thus supporting the treatment direction. Although the SOAP format will not assure good problem-solving skills, it does provide a useful framework within which good problem solving is more likely to occur (Griffith & Ignatavicius, 1986). Thus, the intent of SOAP notes is multifaceted: to improve the quality and continuity of client services, to enhance communication among mental health professionals, to facilitate the counselor in recalling the details of each client's case, and to generate an ongoing assessment of both the client's progress and treatment successes (Kettenbach, 1995; Weed, 1968).

USING THE SOAP NOTE FORMAT

There are four components to SOAP notes. Data collection is divided into two parts: (S) subjective and (O) objective.

The subjective component contains information about the problem from the client's perspective and that of significant others, whereas the objective information consists of those observations made by the counselor. The assessment section demonstrates how the subjective and the objective data are being formulated, interpreted, and reflected upon, and the plan section summarizes the treatment direction. What follows is a description of the content for each section of the SOAP notes, a brief clinical scenario with an example of how this approach might be written, and a short list of "rules" to remember when writing case notes.

Subjective

The data-gathering section of the SOAP format is probably the most troublesome to write because it is sometimes difficult to determine what constitutes subjective and objective content. The subjective portion of the SOAP notes contains information told to the counselor. In this section the client's feelings, concerns, plans or goals, and thoughts, plus the intensity of the problem(s) and its impact on significant relationships in the client's life are recorded. Pertinent comments supplied by family members, friends, probation officers, and so forth can also be included in this section. Without losing accuracy, the entry should be as brief and concise as possible; the client's perceptions of the problem(s) should be immediately clear to an outside reader.

It is our opinion that client quotations should be kept to a minimum. First, when quotations are overused they make the record more difficult to review for client themes and to track the effectiveness of therapeutic interventions. Second, when reviewed by outside readers such as peer review panels, audit committees, or by a client's attorney, the accuracy and integrity of the notes might be called into question. According to Hart, Berndt, and Caramazza (1985), the number of *verbatim* bits of information an individual is able to retain is quite small, 2 to 20 bits, with most estimates at the lower end. Other research suggests that information retained in short-term memory is only briefly held, 30 seconds to a few minutes at best, unless a very conscious effort is made to retain it (see Anderson & Bowers, 1973; Bechtel & Abrahamsen, 1990). This means that at the close of an hour-long counseling session, unless a quote is taken directly from an audio- or videotaped session, it is very unlikely that someone could accurately remember much information verbatim. In short, given this research, it seems a prudent practice to keep the use of quotations to a minimum.

If and when quotations are used, the counselor should record only key words or a very brief phrase. This might include client words indicating suicidal or homicidal ideation, a major shift in the client's well-being, nonconforming behaviors, or statements suggesting a compromise in the type and quality of care the client will receive, such as when a client is unwilling or fails to provide necessary information. Quotations might also be used to document inappropriately aggressive or abusive language toward the counselor that seems threatening. Comments suggesting a potentially lethal level of "denial" should be documented. For instance, a father accused of shaking his 6-month-old daughter when she would not stop crying says, "I only scared her when I shook her, I didn't hurt her." Because the child's life might be in jeopardy should the father repeat his behavior, his comments need to be recorded. For example, the counselor might write: "Minimizes the effects of shaking infant daughter. States, 'I only scared her.'"

It is also important to document statements that suggest the client may be confused as to time, place, or person, or if he or she is experiencing a sudden change in mental status stability or level of functioning. For example, if during the session the client suddenly seems disoriented and unable to track the conversation, this information needs to be noted. To assess the client's mental status, the counselor might ask the client the name of the current U.S. president. If the client responds incorrectly, this discrepancy should be noted in quotations within the client file.

Finally, a client's negative or positive change in attitude toward counseling should be chronicled because it serves as a marker in the assessment of counseling effectiveness. A statement such as "Therapy is really helping me put my life into perspective" could be written as "Reports 'therapy is really helping.'" This information is especially important if the client was initially resistant to therapy. The goal is not to give a verbatim account of what the client says, but rather to reflect current areas of client concern and to support or validate the counselor's interpretations and interventions in the assessment and plan sections of the SOAP notes.

Given the open nature of client files to other health care professionals and paraprofessionals (e.g., certain managed care personnel), the counselor should be mindful of the type of client and family information included in the client's record. Unless insidious family life and political, religious, and racial views are the focus of the problem(s), secondary details of such views should be omitted (Eggland, 1988; Philpott, 1986). The counselor should not repeat inflammatory statements critical of other health care professionals or the quality of services provided because these comments may compromise the client's care by antagonizing the staff or might be interpreted as malicious or damaging to the reputation of another. Rather than using the names of specific people when recording the session, the counselor might use general words such as a "fellow employee" or "mental health worker," and briefly and concisely report the themes of the client's complaint(s). In addition, the names of others in the life of the client are typically unnecessary to record. It is important to remember that the names the client mentions during counseling (with few exceptions) are not a legitimate part of the client's care and, as such, should be omitted from the client's file.

The content in the subjective section belongs to the client, unless otherwise noted. For brevity's sake, the counselor should simply write, "reports, states, says, describes, indicates, complains of," and so on, in place of "The client says." For instance, instead of writing, "Today the client says 'I am experiencing much more trouble at home—in my marriage—much more marital trouble since the time before our last

session,'" the counselor might write "client reports increased marital problems since last session." Also, because it is implied that the counselor is the writer of the entry, it is not necessary for the counselor to refer to himself or herself, unless it is necessary to avoid confusion.

Objective

In a word, the "objective" portion of the SOAP format should be factual. It is written in quantifiable terms—that which can be seen, heard, smelled, counted, or measured. There are two types of objective data: the counselor's observations and outside written materials. Counselor observations include any physical, interpersonal, or psychological findings that the counselor witnesses. This could consist of the client's general appearance, affect and behavior, the nature of the therapeutic relationship, and the client's strengths. When appropriate, this might include the client's mental status, ability to participate in counseling, and his or her responses to the process. If they are available, outside written materials such as reports from other counselors/therapists, the results of psychological tests, or medical records can also be included in this section.

The counselor's findings are stated in precise and descriptive terms. Words that act to modify the content of the objective observations, such as "appeared" or "seemed" should be avoided. If the counselor feels hesitant in making a definitive observational statement, adequate justification for the reluctance should be provided. The phrase *as evidenced by* is helpful in these situations. For example, one day the client arrives and is almost lethargic in her responses and has difficulty tracking the flow of the session. This behavior is markedly different from previous sessions in which the client was very engaged in the counseling process. When questioned, the client denies feeling depressed. In recording this observation, the counselor might chart, "Appeared depressed, as evidenced by significantly less verbal exchange; intermittent difficulty tracking. Hair uncombed; clothes unkempt. Denies feeling depressed."

When recording observations, counselors should avoid labels, personal judgments, value-laden language, or opinionated statements (i.e., personal opinion rather than professional opinion). Words that may have a negative connotation, such as "uncooperative," "manipulative," "abusive," "obnoxious," "normal," "spoiled," "dysfunctional," "functional," and "drunk," are open to personal interpretation. Instead, record observed behaviors, allowing future readers to draw their own conclusions. For example, one should not record, "Client arrived drunk to this session and was rude, obnoxious, and uncooperative." Instead, one should simply record what is seen, heard, or smelled, for example: Consider, "Client smelled of alcohol; speech slow and deliberate in nature; uncontrollable giggles even after stumbling against door jam; unsteady gait."

Assessment

The assessment section is essentially a summarization of the counselor's *clinical thinking* regarding the client's problem(s). The assessment section serves to synthesize and analyze the data from the subjective and objective portions of the notes. The assessment is generally stated in the form of a psychiatric diagnosis based on the *Diagnostic and Statistical Manual of Mental Disorders*, text revision (*DSM-IV-TR*; American Psychiatric Association, 2000) and is included in every entry. Although some counselors resist the idea of labeling their clients with a *DSM-IV-TR* diagnosis, third-party payers and accrediting bodies such as the Joint Commission on Accreditation of Hospitals require that this be done. According to Ginter and Glauser (2001), "Ignorance of the *DSM* system is not congruent with current expectations concerning counseling practice" (p. 70).

The assessment section can also include *clinical impressions* (i.e., a conclusion lacking full support) that are used to "rule out" and "rule in" a diagnosis. In more complex cases, in which insufficient information exists to support a particular diagnosis, clinical impressions work much like a decision tree, helping the counselor to systematically arrive at his or her conclusions. More important, when clinical impressions are used and stated, they enable outside reviewers and other health professionals to follow the counselor's reasoning in selecting the client's final diagnosis and treatment direction. When writing clinical impressions, counselors should identify them as such. For the sake of clarity, the relevant points from the data sections should be summarized. Doing this will assist the counselor in formalizing a tentative diagnosis and will demonstrate to outside reviewers the sequence of logic used to arrive at the final diagnosis.

There is debate regarding the use of clinical impressions. Piazza and Baruth (1990) and Snider (1987) recommended against their use, whereas Mitchell (1991) viewed the use of clinical impressions as a powerful entry. In place of clinical impressions, some counselors keep personal or shadow notes. These notes are kept separate from the client's file, and the counselor uses them to record tentative impressions (Keith-Spiegel & Koocher, 1995; Thompson, 1990). This practice needs to be carefully reconsidered. The logistics of maintaining a separate set of notes are almost nightmarish, given the quantity of documentation required in most mental health clinics. Also, there are serious legal and ethical considerations. For the protection of the practitioner, client records need to demonstrate the counselor's thinking and reasoning regarding the diagnosis selected and the elimination of other possible diagnoses (Swenson, 1993). Even though a counselor's set of personal or shadow notes may be subpoenaed by the courts, by recording separate sets of notes the client's record can lack a logical progression of evaluation, planning, and treatment of the problem(s). This leaves the counselor "with no evidence of competence when a lawsuit happens" (Swenson, 1993, p. 162). Simply stated, we believe that one set of notes should be kept and that it is appropriate to incorporate clinical impressions in the record.

An example of the appropriate use of clinical impressions is as follows. A counselor working in a family services agency is assessing a 7-year-old child who has been referred for possible attention-deficit/hyperactivity disorder. The report

from the child's teacher describes the child as being unable to stay on tasks for longer than 5 minutes, being frequently out of his chair, and not seeming to respect other children's needs for "personal space." When the case history is taken, the child's mother provides the information that there were times when she drank frequently and excessively, sometimes to the point of "blacking out," and the mother recalls that this "may have occurred" during the first trimester of her pregnancy. Although there is insufficient information with which to make a diagnosis, a reasonable clinical impression related to a tentative diagnosis is to "rule out fetal alcohol syndrome/effects (FAS/FAE)." Although the counselor is unable to make a definitive diagnosis, given the child's prenatal history, current level of hyperactivity, and decreased attention span, an entry subtitled "Clinical impression: Rule out FAS/FAE" clearly demonstrates the counselor's understanding of childhood psychopathology and developmental issues and supports a referral to a neurological team for evaluation. If the evaluation confirms FAS/FAE, this will determine the diagnosis rendered and the treatment direction.

The assessment portion of the SOAP notes is the most likely section to be read by others, such as outside reviewers auditing records. When making a diagnosis, the counselor needs to ask the question, "Are there adequate data here to support the client diagnosis?" If sufficient data have been collected, the subjective and the objective sections should reasonably support the clinical diagnosis. However, if the counselor is feeling uncomfortable or unsure regarding the accuracy of the diagnosis, this ambivalence might suggest that insufficient data have been collected or that a consultation with a senior colleague is in order.

Plan

The last portion of the SOAP notes is the plan. This section could be described as the parameters of counseling interventions used. The plan generally consists of two parts: the action plan and the prognosis. Information contained under the action plan includes the date of the next appointment, the interventions used during the session, educational instruction (if it was given), treatment progress, and the treatment direction for the next session.

Sometimes clients will benefit from a multiagency or multidisciplinary team approach. When such referrals are made, the names and agencies to which the client was referred are recorded (names involved in the referral should be recorded). If the counselor believes that a consultation is needed, it is documented in this section and includes the telephone contacts made to the consultant regarding the client.

The client prognosis is recorded in the plan section. The prognosis is a forecast of the probable gains to be made by the client given the diagnosis, the client's personal resources, and motivation to change. Generally, progress assessments are described in terms such as *poor, guarded, fair, good,* or *excellent,* followed by supporting reasons for the particular prognosis. The plan section brings the SOAP notes and the treatment direction full circle. Table 1 summarizes the SOAP noting format and provides examples for the reader.

A Summarization of SOAP Definitions and Examples

Section	Definitions	Examples
Subjective (S)	What the client tells you What pertinent others tell you about the client Basically, how the client experiences the world	Client's feelings, concerns, plans, goals, and thoughts Intensity of problems and impact on relationships Pertinent comments by family, case managers, behavioral therapists, etc. Client's orientation to time, place, and person Client's verbalized changes toward helping
Objective (O)	Factual What the counselor personally observes/witnesses Quantifiable: what was seen, counted, smelled, heard, or measured Outside written materials received	The client's general appearance, affect, behavior Nature of the helping relationship Client's demonstrated strengths and weaknesses Test results, materials from other agencies, etc., are to be noted and attached.
Assessment (A)	Summarizes the counselor's clinical thinking A synthesis and analysis of the subjective and objective portion of the notes	For counselor: Include clinical diagnosis and clinical impressions (if any). For care providers: How would you label the client's behavior and the reasons (if any) for this behavior?
Plan (P)	Describes the parameters of treatment Consists of an action plan and prognosis	Action plan: Include interventions used, treatment progress, and direction. Counselors should include the date of next appointment. Prognosis: Include the anticipated gains from the interventions.

SCENARIO AND SAMPLE SOAP NOTES

The following is a very brief hypothetical scenario and a sample of how the SOAP notes might be written. Abbreviations have not been used because the use and types of abbreviations vary from institution to institution. *Finally, in this situation the counselor is responsible for the intake session.*

Scenario

Cecil is a 34-year-old man who was mandated by the courts to obtain counseling to resolve his problems with domestic violence. He comes into the office, slams the door, and announces in a loud and irritated voice, "This counseling stuff is crap! There's no parking! My wife and kids are gone! And I gotta pay for something that don't work!"

Throughout most of the counseling session Cecil remains agitated. Speaking in an angry and aggressive voice, he tells you that his probation officer told him he was a good man and could get his wife and kids back. He demands to know why you are not really helping him get back what is most important to him. He insists that "Mary just screws everything up!" He goes on to tell you of a violent argument he and Mary had last night regarding the privileges of their daughter Nicole, who just turned 16. You are aware that there is a restraining order against Cecil.

During the session, you learn Cecil was raised in a physically and verbally abusive family until he was 11, at which time he was placed in protective custody by social services, where he remained until he was 18. He goes on to tell you that he has been arrested numerous times for "brawling" and reports that sometimes the littlest things make him angry and he just explodes, hitting whatever is available—the walls, his wife, the kids, and three guys at work. Cecil also reports

prior arrests for domestic violence. He admits that at various times, he has been both physically and emotionally abusive to Mary and the children but insists that it was needed "to straighten them out." Just before leaving your office, Cecil rushes from his chair and stands within a foot of you. Angrily, with his fists and jaw clenched, he says, "This is the same old B.S. You guys are just all talk." He storms from the room.

Sample SOAP Notes

7/7/01. 2 p.m. (S) Reports counseling is not helping him get his family back. Insists the use of violence has been needed to "straighten out" family members. Reports history of domestic violence. Recent history: States he met and verbally fought with his wife yesterday regarding the privileges of oldest child. Personal history: childhood physical and mental abuse resulting in foster care placement, ages 11–18. (O) Generally agitated throughout the session. Toward the end of the session stood up, with clenched fists and jaw, angrily stated that counseling is "same old B.S.!" Rushed out of office. (A) Physical Abuse of Adult [V61.1, *DSM* code] and Child(ren) [V61.21]. Clinical impressions: Rule out Intermittent Explosive Disorder given bouts of uncontrolled rage with non-specific emotional trigger. (P) Rescheduled for 7/14/01 @ 2 p.m.; prognosis guarded due to low level of motivation to change. Continue cognitive therapy. Refer to Dr. Smith for psychiatric/medication evaluation. Referred to Men's Alternative to Violence Group. Next session, introduce use of "time-outs." S. Cameron, Ph.D., LPCC (signature).

GENERAL GUIDELINES FOR SOAP NOTING

Client records are legal documents. For the most part, in a court of law, they represent the quality of services provided by the counselor (Mitchell, 1991; Scalise, 2000; Thompson, 1990). To ensure both the quality and the accuracy of the notes and to safeguard the integrity of the counselor, the following guidelines should be observed when writing SOAP notes.

Record the session immediately after the session while it is still fresh in your mind. This avoids the uncertainty, confusion, errors, or inaccuracies that are most likely to occur when you try to complete all the files at the day's end. Start each entry with the date (month, day, and year) and time the session began. Make each entry legible and neat with no grammar, spelling, or punctuation errors. Finally, the client record should reflect the counselor's level of training and expertise. For example, the counselor's extensive use of psychoanalytic-based terminology without having received such training may cause other professionals to question the competency of the counselor. The American Counseling Association's (ACA, 1995) Code of Ethics takes a clear position on counselors limiting practice to level of competence, and because records may be reviewed by others, the record's language must be congruent with level of competence. These procedures will alleviate misunderstandings between professionals and minimize the potential of a lawsuit (Swenson, 1993).

All client contact or attempted contact should be recorded using the SOAP format. This includes all telephone calls, messages left on answering machines, or messages left with individuals who answered the phone. Letters that were mailed to the client would be noted in the record along with a photocopy of the signed letter.

When recording a session, keep in mind that altered entries arouse suspicions and can create significant problems for the counselor in a court of law (Norris, 1995). If an error is made, never erase, obliterate, use correction fluid, or in any way attempt to obscure the mistake. Instead, the error should be noted by enclosing it in brackets, drawing a single line through the incorrect word(s), and writing the word "error" above or to the side of the mistake. The counselor should follow this correction with her or his initials, the full date, and time of the correction. The mistake should still be readable, indicating the counselor is only attempting to clarify the mistake not cover it up. If not

typed, all entries should be written in black ballpoint pen, which allows for easy photocopying should the file be requested at a later date. Furthermore, notes should never be written in pencil or felt-tipped pen because pencil can be easily erased or altered, whereas felt-tipped pen is easily smudged or distorted should something spill on the notes.

At the conclusion of the entry, the counselor needs to sign off using a legal signature—generally considered to be the first initial and last name followed by the counselor's title. All entries, regardless of their size, are followed by the counselor's legal signature. There should be no empty space between the content of the SOAP notes and the signature. Blank spaces may later be interpreted (e.g., by a lawyer) to mean that there is missing information or that the counselor failed to provide "complete care" (Norris, 1995); even worse, empty spaces can be filled in by another person without the counselor's knowledge. Writing should be continuous with no lines skipped between entries or additional commentary squeezed in between the lines or in the margins. Table 2 offers readers a quick reference list of "do's and don'ts."

CONCLUSION

In this era of accountability, counselors are expected to use a more systematic approach in documenting rendered services (Ginter & Glauser, in press; Norris, 1995; Scalise, 2000) and demonstrating treatment effectiveness (JCAHO, 2000). Good documentation is a fundamental part of providing minimal client care, and needs to be mastered like any other counseling skill. As the standards for recording receive increased scrutiny by both managed care organizations and the National Committee for Quality Assurance, the importance of documentation has changed "from something that *should* be done well to something that *must* be done well" (Kettenbach, 1995, p. iii), especially if counseling is to survive in this age of managed resources. SOAP notes are a proven and effective means of addressing this new mandate. We hope that this article will help others fulfill this dictate, for there is no substitute for concisely written and well-documented case notes.

TABLE 2

Guidelines for Subjective, Objective, Assessment, Plan (SOAP) Noting

Do	Avoid
Be brief and concise.	Avoid using names of other clients, family members, or others named by client.
Keep quotes to a minimum.	Avoid terms like seems, appears.
Use an active voice.	Avoid value-laden language, common labels, opinionated statements.
Use precise and descriptive terms.	Do not use terminology unless trained to do so.
Record immediately after each session.	Do not erase, obliterate, use correction fluid, or in any way attempt to obscure mistakes.
Start each new entry with date and time of session.	Do not leave blank spaces between entries.
Write legibly and neatly.	Do not try to squeeze additional commentary between lines or in margins.
Use proper spelling, grammar, and punctuation.	
Document all contacts or attempted contacts.	
Use only black ink if notes are handwritten.	
Sign-off using legal signature, plus your title.	

Cameron and turtle-song

REFERENCES

American Counseling Association. (1995). *ACA code of ethics and standards of practice*. Alexandria, VA: Author.

American Psychiatric Association. (2000). *Diagnostic and statistical manual of mental disorders* (Text rev.). Washington, DC: Author.

Anderson, J., & Bowers, G. (1973). *Human association memory*. Washington, DC: Winston.

Bechtel, W., & Abrahamsen, A. (1990). *Connectionism and the mind: Introduction to parallel processing in networks*. Cambridge, MA: Basil Blackwell.

Eggland, E. T. (1988). Charting: How and why to document your care daily—and fully. *Nursing, 18*(11), 76–84.

Ginter, E. J., & Glauser, A. (2001). Effective use of the *DSM* from a developmental/wellness perspective. In E. R. Welfel & R. E. Ingersoll (Eds.), *The mental health desk reference* (pp. 69–77). New York: Wiley.

Griffith, J., & Ignatavicius, D. (1986). *The writer's handbook: The complete guide to clinical documentation, professional writing and research papers*. Baltimore: Resource Applications.

Hart, J., Berndt, R., & Caramazza, A. (1985, August). Category specific naming deficit following cerebral infractions. *Nature, 316*, 339–340.

Joint Commission on Accreditation of Healthcare Organizations. (2000). *Consolidated standards manual for child, adolescent, and adult psychiatric, alcoholism, and drug abuse facilities*. Chicago: Author.

Keith-Spiegel, P., & Koocher, G. P. (1995). *Ethics in psychology: Professional standards and cases*. New York: Random House.

Kettenbach, G. (1995). *Writing SOAP notes*. Philadelphia: Davis.

Mitchell, R. W. (1991). *The ACA Legal Series: Documentation in counseling records* (Vol. 2). Alexandria, VA: American Counseling Association.

Norris, J. (1995). *Mastering documentation*. Springhouse, PA: Springhouse.

Philpott, M. (1986). Twenty rules for good charting. *Nursing, 16*(8), 63.

Piazza, N. J., & Baruth, N. E. (1990). Client record guidelines. *Journal of Counseling & Development, 68*, 313–316.

Ryback, R. S. (1974). *The problem oriented record in psychiatry and mental health care*. New York: Grune & Stratton.

Scalise, J. J. (1999). The ethical practice of marriage and family therapy. In A. Horne (Ed.), *Family counseling and therapy* (3rd ed., pp. 565–596). Itasca, IL: Peacock.

Shaw, M. (1997). *Charting made incredibly easy*. Springhouse, PA: Springhouse.

Siegal, C., & Fischer, S. K. (1981). *Psychiatric records in mental health*. New York: Brunner/Mazel.

Snider, P. D. (1987). Client records: Inexpensive liability protection for mental health counselors. *Journal of Mental Health Counseling, 9*, 134–141.

Swenson, L. C. (1993). *Psychology and law for the helping professions*. Pacific Grove, CA: Brooks/Cole.

Thompson, A. (1990). *Guide to ethical practice in psychotherapy*. New York: Wiley.

Weed, L. L. (1964). Medical records, patient care and medical education. *Irish Journal of Medical Education, 6*, 271–282.

Weed, L. L. (1968). Medical records that guide and teach. *New England Journal of Medicine, 278*, 593–600, 652–657.

Weed, L. L. (1971). Quality control and the medical record. *Archive of Internal Medicine, 127*, 101–105.

References

Preface

Footnote:

1   http://www.stfm.org/fmhub/Fullpdf/Jan00/re1.pdf (as of July 09)

Endnote:

1   Pert,C. (1997), *Molecules of Emotion*, New York, NY., Scribner, p.223

Chapter 1

1   Pierce, B. (2007) 'The Use of Biofield Therapies in Cancer Care', *Clinical Journal of Oncology Nursing*, April; 11(2) pp. 253-258

2   http://www.newton.ac.uk/newlife.html (assessed May 2009)

3   M. Talbot, *Holographic Universe* (New York: Harper Perennial, 1992), p.46

4   http://www.insightcenter.net/where-psychology-meets-physics/the-implicate-order/ (assessed May 2009)

5   M. Talbot, *Holographic Universe*, (New York: Harper Perennial, 1992) p. 47

6   D Chopra, M/D, *Quantum Healing: exploring the frontiers of mind/body medicine*, Bantam Books New York, NY(1990) p. 15

7   C. Pert, *Molecules of Emotion* Scribner New York, NY, 1997, p.276

8   McCraty, R. PhD, Atkinson. M. Tomasino, D. BA and Tiller, W. A. PhD. The Electricity of Touch: Detection and Measurement of Cardiac Exchange Between People, In: Karl H. Pribram, ed. Brain and Values: Is a Biological Science of Values Possible. Mahwah, NJ: Lawrence Erlbaum Associates, Publishers, 1998: 359-379.

9   William A.Tiller, *Science and Human Transformation* (Pavior

Publishing,CA 1997), p.14-15

10　The Upledger Institute, Inc., brochure Rev. 09/00

11　C. Pert, *Molecules of Emotion* Scribner New York, NY, 1997, p.276

12　http://www.ncbi.nlm.nih.gov/pubmed/1299456　(assessed May 2009)

13　Interview by William Lee Rand with James L. Oschman, Ph.D., *Reiki News Magazine*, Vol. One, Issue Three, Winter 2002. ©2002 Vision Publications.

Chapter 2

Foot note for chapter 2

1　Peptide: any of various natural or synthetic compounds containing two or more amino acids linked by the carboxyl group of one amino acid and the amino group of another. Candace Pert, *Molecules of Emotion*, (Scribner, 1997), p. 352

2　Neuropeptide: any of the nearly 100small peptide informational substances initially described as neuronalsecretions. Ibid, p. 351

3　Ligands: any of a variety of small molecules that specifically bind to a cellular receptor and in so doing convey an informational message to the cell. Ibid, p. 350

Endnotes

1　J.Crellin, F. Ania, *Professionalism & Ethics in Complementary and Alternative Medicine*, Hawthorn Press Inc, Binghamton, NY 2002, p. 54

2　Snyder L (ed) *Complementary and Alternative Medicine(Ethics, the Patient, and the Physician)*, Humana Press Inc., Totowa, NJ 2007, p 15

3　C. Pert, *Molecules of Emotion*, Scribner, New York, NY 1997, p 282

4　J.Crellin, F. Ania, *Professionalism & Ethics in Complementary and Alternative Medicine*, Hawthorn Press Inc, Binghamton,

NY 2002, p 56

5   http://www.rainforestinfo.org.au/background/rainfwld.htm
    (assessed May 2009)

6   http://www.rainforestinfo.org.au/background/rainfwld.htm
    (assessed May 2009)

7   A. Lockie, Dr., *The Family Guide to Homeopathy*,
    Fireside/Simon & Schuster Inc., New York, NY., 1993, p. 190

8   http://www.tstcm.com/html/course_desc.htm?dep_id=1&
    crs_id=2 (assessed June 2009)

9   Snyder L (ed) *Complementary and Alternative Medicine(Ethics,
    the Patient, and the Physician)*, Humana Press Inc., Totowa, NJ
    2007, p 23

10 Ibid., p. 40

11 http://www.pbs.org/wgbh/nova/doctors/oath_modern.html
    (assessed May 2009)

12 D Chopra, M/D, *Quantum Healing: exploring the frontiers of
    mind/body medicine*, Bantam Books New York, NY(1990)
    preface

13 J. Oschman, *Energy Medicine in Therapeuics and Human
    Performance*, Butterworth-Heinemann/Elsevier, Philadelphia,
    PA, 2003, p. 282

14 C. Pert, *Molecules of Emotion*, Scribner, New York, NY 1997,
    p147

15 Ibid., 145

16 A. Wise, *Awakening the Mind*, Tarcher/Penguin Putnam Inc,
    New York, NY, 2002 back jacket cover

17 Ibid., pgs 9-13

18 D Chopra, M/D, *Quantum Healing: exploring the frontiers of
    mind/body medicine*, Bantam Books New York, NY(1990) p
    175

19 Ibid.

20 Ibid, p.176

21 C. Pert, *Molecules of Emotion*, Scribner, New York, NY 1997, p
    2473

22 Ibid., p. 242

23 Ibid., p. 306

Chapter 3

1. Berman JD, Straus SE Implementing a research agenda for complementary and alternative medicine. *Annual Review of Medicine.* 2004:55:239-254

2   Simon Y Mills, Regulation in complementary and alternative medicine, Research coordinatior, Complementary Health Studies Programme, Department of Lifelong Learning, School of Education, Exeter EX1 2LU
BMJ. 2001 January 20;322(7279): 158-160
PMCID:PMC1119419

3   Gerard Bodeker and Gemma Burford (eds), *Traditional, complementary and alternative medicine: policy and public health perspectives.* Publisher Imperial College Press, London, 2007
ISBN 978-1-86094-646-5

4   http://www.who.int/bulletin/volumes/86/1/07-046458/en /index.html (assessed May 2009)

5   http://incamresearch.ca/index.php?id=40,0,0,1,0,0 &menu=0 (assessed May 2009)

6   http://nccam.nih.gov/research/clinicaltrials/factsheet/clini caltrials.pdf (asssessed May 2009)

7   M. Beauregard,PhD D. O'Leary, *The Spiritual Brain: A neuro-scientis's case for the existence of the soul,* Harper One,New York, NY, 2007 p.xv

8   C. Pert, *Molecules of Emotion* Scribner New York, NY, 1997, p.105

9   Snyder L (ed) *Complementary and Alternative Medicine(Ethics, the Patient, and the Physician),* Humana Press Inc., Totowa, NJ 2007, p.80

10 http://www.brighton.ac.uk/ncor/osteo_research/EBP_tuto rial_case_report.pdf (assessed August 2009)

11 http://www.thebodyworker.com/businesssoapnotes.html

(assessed February 2010)

Chapter 4

Footnote from Chaper 4 page 1:

1   Nahin, RL, Barnes PM, Stussman BJ, and Bloom B. Costs of Complementary and Alternative Medicine (CAM) and Frequency of Visits to CAM Practitioners: United States, 2007. National health statistics reports; no 18. Hyattsville, MD: National Center for Health Statistics. 2009

2   Office of the Actuary, Centers for Medicare and Medicaid Services, National Health Expenditure Data for 2007. U.S. Department of Health and Human Services. Available at: http://www.cms.hhs.gov/NationalHealthExpendData/02_N ationalHealthAccountsHistorical.asp#TopOfPage. Accessed June 25, 2009

3   Barnes PM, Bloom B, Nahin RL. Complementary and Alternative Medicine Use Among Adults and Children: United States, 2007. National health statistics reports; no 12. Hyattsville, MD: National Center for Health Statistics. 2008.

Endnotes

1   Snyder L (ed) *Complementary and Alternative Medicine(Ethics, the Patient, and the Physician)*, Humana Press Inc., Totowa, NJ 2007, p. 84

2   Ibid., p.13

3   Eisenberg, DM. Advising patients who seek alternative medical therapies. Ann Intern Med 1997;127(1):61-69

4   http://www.hprac.org (as of July 2009)

5   http://www.hprac.org/en/about/mandate.asp (as of July 2009)

6   Snyder L (ed) *Complementary and Alternative Medicine(Ethics, the Patient, and the Physician)*, Humana Press Inc., Totowa, NJ 2007, p.8

7   Ibid., p. 147

8   J. Crellin, F. Ania, *Professionalism & Ethics in Complementary and Alternative Medicine*, Binghamton, NY: Haworth Press Inc. 2002, p 61

9   Ibid., p. 28

10 Ibid., p. 145

11 Ibid,, p. 101

12 Snyder L (ed) *Complementary and Alternative Medicine(Ethics, the Patient, and the Physician)*, Humana Press Inc., Totowa, NJ 2007, p. 107

13 Ibid., p. 104

14 Hospice Palliative Care Ontario (HPCO), 2011 Hospice Palliative Care Conference April 10-12, 2011 2 Carlton Street, Suite 707, Toronto, ON M5B 1J3

15 Canadian Federation of Independent Business D-IN0530-0312(213) http://www.cfib.ca/legis/national/pdf/5198.pdf (as of May 2009)

16 http://www.e-laws.gov.on.ca/html/statutes/english/elaws_statutes_96h02_e.htm (as of May 2009)

17 Ibid.,

18 J. Crellin, F. Ania, *Professionalism & Ethics in Complementary and Alternative Medicine*, Binghamton, NY: Haworth Press Inc. 2002, p. 154

19 http://nccam.nih.gov/health/reiki/ (as of May 2009)

20 Jonas, W.B., Crawford, C.C., *Healing, Intention, and Energy Medicine*, (Elsevier Ltd., 2003) Philadelphia PA p.179

21 http://www.intlacademy.com/dresscodepolicy.htm(as of June 2009)

22 http://wiki.answers.com/Q/What_are_some_examples_of_pathogenic_diseases_and_how_can_they_be_treated_and_controlled (as of June 2009)

23 http://www.iaff.org/hs/Resi/infdis/What_are_the_routes_of_exposure.htm (as of June2009)

24 http://www.iaff.org/hs/Resi/infdis/What_is_an_airborne_disease.htm (as of June2009)

25 http://meds.queensu.ca/postgraduate/policies/blood_borne_ diseases (as of June2009)

26 http://www.iaff.org/hs/Resi/infdis/What_is_a_bloodborne_d isease.htm (as of June2009)

27 http://www.iaff.org/he/Resi/infdis/What_are_the_modes_ of_transmission.htm (as of June 2009)

28 http://www.iaff.org/hs/Resi/infdis/What_is_Hepatitis_A_ .htm (as of June2009)

29 http://www.iaff.org/hs/Resi/infdis/What_is_Hepatitis_B_ .htm (as of June2009)

30 http://www.iaff.org/hs/Resi/infdis/What_is_Hepatitis_C .htm (as of June2009)

31 http://www.cdc.gov/hepatitis/index.htm (as of June2009)

32 http://www.iaff.org/hs/Resi/infdis/What_is_HIV_AIDS_ .htm (as of June2009)

33 http://www.cdc.gov/hiv/topics/basic/index.htm (as of June 2009)

34 Control of Communicable Diseases Manual edited by James B. Chin, APHA, 2000 ect

Chapter 5

Footnote to Chapter 5 page 1

1   Nihon Iji Shinpo (a medical journal with the title of "Japanese Medical News")

Endnote

1   F A Petter, *Reiki the Legacy of Dr. Usui,* (Lotus Light- Shangri- La, Twin Lakes, WI) 1998 p 17-18

Chapter 6

1   Hospice Simcoe, *Visiting Volunteer Training Manual,* (self published 2004 p. 16-28)

2   http://scrubnotes.blogspot.com/2007/08/how-to-write-histo ryphysical-or-soap.html (as of Jan2010)

3   http://metaot.com/notes-SOAP (as of Feb 2010)

4   The Military and Hospitaller Order of Saint Lazarus of Jerusalem &Canadian Hospice Palliative Care Association, *A Caregiver's Guide*, (self published 2004) p. 163

5   http://www.nlm.nih.gov/medlineplus/ency/article/000205.htm (as of July 2009)

6   http://www.nlm.nih.gov/medlineplus/ency/article/000147.htm (as of July 2009)

7   http://www.nlm.nih.gov/medlineplus/ency/article/001265.htm (as of July 2009)

8   http://www.nlm.nih.gov/medlineplus/ency/article/000457.htm (as of July 2009)

9   http://www.nlm.nih.gov/medlineplus/ency/article/000205.htm (as of July 2009)

10   http://www.nlm.nih.gov/medlineplus/ency/article/000066.htm (as of July 2009)

11   http://www.nlm.nih.gov/medlineplus/neurologicdiseases.html (as of July 2009)

12   http://www.nlm.nih.gov/medlineplus/ency/article/001289.htm (as of July 2009)

13   Hospice Simcoe, *Visiting Volunteer Training Manual,* (self published 2004) p 65

14   http://www.canadianpaincoalition.ca/index.php/en/help-centre/conquering-pain/effects-of-pain (as of July 2009)

15   http://www.canadianpaincoalition.ca/index.php/en/help-centre/conquering-pain/all-pain-the-same (as of July 2009)

16   http://www.canadianpaincoalition.ca/index.php/en/help-centre/conquering-pain/talk-to-healthcare-professionals (as of July 2009)

17   http://www.hcpro.com/content/234958.doc (as of July 2009)

18   http://en.wikipedia.org/wiki/Pain_scale (as of July 2009)

19   Feinstein, D. PhD.; Eden, D. Six Pillars of Energy Medicine: Clinical Strengths of a Complementary Paradigm. Alternative Therapies, Jan/Feb 2008, vol. 14. No. 1 p 52

Appendix 3

1   From the Beth Israel Department of Family Medicine, Albert
     Einstein College of Medicine (Dr Kligler); the Department of
     Family Medicine, University of Washington (Dr Gordon);
     the Department of Family Medicine, UMDNJ-RWJ Medical
     School (Dr Stuart); and the Department of Family Medicine,
     University of Texas Medical Branch at Galveston (Dr
     Sierpina).

AYNI
BOOKS

"Ayni" is a Quechua word meaning "reciprocity" – sharing, giving and receiving - whatever you give out comes back to you. To be in Ayni is to be in balance, harmony and right relationship with oneself and nature, of which we are all an intrinsic part. Complementary and Alternative approaches to health and well-being essentially follow a holistic model, within which one is given support and encouragement to move towards a state of balance, true health and wholeness, ultimately leading to the awareness of one's unique place in the Universal jigsaw of life – Ayni, in fact.